Neurocritical Care Nursing Management of Stroke

Editor

WANDRIA DALLAS

CRITICAL CARE NURSING CLINICS OF NORTH AMERICA

www.ccnursing.theclinics.com

Consulting Editor
DEBORAH GARBEE

March 2023 • Volume 35 • Number 1

ELSEVIER

1600 John F. Kennedy Boulevard • Suite 1800 • Philadelphia, Pennsylvania, 19103-2899

http://www.theclinics.com

CRITICAL CARE NURSING CLINICS OF NORTH AMERICA Volume 35, Number 1
March 2023 ISSN 0899-5885, ISBN-13: 978-0-443-18326-3

Editor: Kerry Holland
Developmental Editor: Ann Gielou M. Posedio

Critical Care Nursing Clinics of North America (ISSN 0899-5885) is published quarterly by Elsevier Inc., 360 Park Avenue South, New York, NY 10010-1710. Months of issue are March, June, September, and December. Business and Editorial Offices: 1600 John F. Kennedy Blvd., Suite 1800, Philadelphia, PA 19103-2899. Periodicals postage paid at New York, NY and additional mailing offices. Subscription prices are $160.00 per year for US individuals, $456.00 per year for US institutions, $100.00 per year for US students and residents, $206.00 per year for Canadian individuals, $573.00 per year for Canadian institutions, $230.00 per year for international individuals, $573.00 per year for international institutions, $115.00 per year for international students/residents and $100.00 per year for Canadian students/residents. To receive student/resident rate, orders must be accompanied by name of affiliated institution, data of term, and the *signature* of program/residency coordinator on institution letterhead. Orders will be billed at individual rate until proof of status is received. Foreign air speed delivery is included in all *Clinics* subscription prices. All prices are subject to change without notice. **POSTMASTER:** Send address changes to *Critical Care Nursing Clinics of North America*, Elsevier Health Sciences Division, Subscription Customer Service, 3251 Riverport Lane, Maryland Heights, MO 63043. **Customer Service: 1-800-654-2452 (US and Canada); 314-447-8871 (outside US and Canada). Fax: 314-447-8029. E-mail:** JournalsCustomerService-usa@elsevier.com **(for print support)** and JournalsOnlineSupport-usa@elsevier.com **(for online support).**

Reprints. For copies of 100 or more of articles in this publication, please contact the Commercial Reprints Department, Elsevier Inc., 360 Park Avenue South, New York, New York, 10010-1710; Tel.: 212-633-3874, Fax: 212-633-3820, and E-mail: reprints@elsevier.com.

Critical Care Nursing Clinics of North America is covered in *MEDLINE/PubMed (Index Medicus), International Nursing Index, Nursing Citation Index, Cumulative Index to Nursing and Allied Health Literature, and RNdex Top 100.*

Contributors

CONSULTING EDITOR

DEBORAH GARBEE, PhD, APRN, ACNS-BC, FCNS
Associate Dean for Professional Practice, Community Service and Advanced Nursing Practice, Professor of Clinical Nursing, Louisiana State University Health Sciences Center New Orleans School of Nursing, New Orleans, Louisiana

EDITOR

WANDRIA DALLAS, MN, APRN, AGCNS-BC
Clinical Nurse Specialist, Vascular Neurology, Ochsner Louisiana State University Health Shreveport, Shreveport, Louisiana

AUTHORS

CYNTHIA CIMINI, RN, BSN, CCRN, SCRN
Rapides Regional Medical Center, Alexandria, Louisiana

KIMBERLY GLASER, MN, APRN, AGACNP-BC, CCRN
The University of Texas Southwestern Medical Center, William P. Clements Jr. University Hospital, Dallas, Texas

CAREY HECK, PhD, CRNP, AGACNP-BC, CNRN
Associate Professor, Director, Adult-Gerontology Acute Care Nurse Practitioner Program, Thomas Jefferson University, Philadelphia, Pennsylvania

GEMI E. JANNOTTA, PhD, APRN
Department of Anesthesia and Pain Medicine, University of Washington, Seattle, Washington

SARAH L. LIVESAY, DNP, APRN, FNCS, FAAN
Department of Anesthesia and Pain Medicine, University of Washington, Rush University College of Nursing, Seattle, Washington

KRISTINE M. McGLENNEN, DNP, APRN
Department of Anesthesia and Pain Medicine, University of Washington, Seattle, Washington

SHAWN MOREAU, MSN, TCRN, CEN
Rapides Regional Medical Center, Alexandria, Louisiana

HELEN P. NEIL, RN, MSN-HCSM, CLNC, FCN
Louisiana State University Health New Orleans, School of Nursing, New Orleans, Louisiana

PAMELA POURCIAU, MSN, NP-C, SCRN, NC-BC
East Jefferson Neurological Associates, Metairie, Louisiana

BAPPADITYA RAY, MBBS, MD
The University of Texas Southwestern Medical Center, Associate Professor, Department of Neurology and Neurological Surgery (Neurocritical Care Division), Dallas, Texas

BRITTA C. SMITH, DNP, FNP-C
East Jefferson Neurological Associates, Metairie, Louisiana

NICOLE THOMAS, DNP, RN, CCM
Instructor of Clinical Nursing, Louisiana State University Health Science Center School of Nursing, Gonzales, Louisiana

SHAVONNE WILLIAMS, MN, APRN, ACNS-BC, ANVP-BC, SCRN, CCRN-K
Texas Health Presbyterian Hospital, Dallas, Texas

Contents

> Stroke is a leading cause of long-term disability and fifth leading cause of death. Acute ischemic stroke, intracerebral hemorrhage, and subarachnoid hemorrhage, the 3 subtypes of strokes, have varying treatment modalities. Common themes in management advocate for early interventions to reduce morbidity and mortality but not all perception is supported through randomized controlled trials. Each stroke subtype has varying premorbid-related and ictus-related outcome predictive models that have differing sensitivities and specificities.

> Managing risk for aspiration in the stroke patient will assist to decrease one of the major complications that these patients experience, which is post-stroke pneumonia. Using an evidenced-based dysphagia protocol is shown to reduce mortality, morbidity, and length of stay caused by post-stroke pneumonia. Physicians, nurses, speech pathologists, and dieticians will be instrumental in performing ongoing assessments and aspiration-prevention strategies to improve stroke patient outcome and reduce complications. Education, and measurement of comprehension, of the care team, patient, and family concerning dysphagia management and prevention of aspiration pneumonia will assist in achieving the aforementioned goals.

> Hypertension affects 1 in 3 Americans and results in nearly 900,000 inpatient admits annually due to ineffective management. As a primary factor in the development of strokes, hypertension management is essential. The approach to effectively manage hypertension should be done from a multi-point approach to ensure the specific elements that impede the effective management of hypertension within various patient populations are addressed accordingly, which includes, personal, physical, and health needs. The robust implementation of lifestyle modifications, medication therapy, and self-efficacy interventions can improve hypertension management by almost 37%.

> Fever is common in patients with stroke and is associated with worse outcomes. Studies in brain injury informed interventions commonly termed therapeutic temperature management (TTM) to improve the monitoring and management of fever. While the role and benefit of TTM in stroke patients has not been well studied, the nurse and healthcare team must extrapolate existing data to determine how to best monitor and apply TTM after stroke. Nurses should be knowledgeable about interventions to monitor and manage complications of TTM (eg, shivering), the studies underway to quantify the impact of fever treatment and emerging technology expected to improve TTM.

> Since the intial outbreak of the coronavirus-2019 (COVID-19) in December 2019, a variety of neurologic manifestations have been linked to this virus, including stroke. Comprehensive review of worldwide studies using various methodologies indicated a correlation of increased stroke risk in patients with COVID-19. The literature reivew also revealed increased morbidity and mortality among patients with COVID-19 and stroke as compared to those with only stroke. This pandemic, with its related healthcare staffing shortages, revealed the requisite to utilize innovative technologies such as Tele-Neurology, as well as public health campaigns focusing on stroke recognition and early treatment.

> Decompressive hemicraniectomy (DHC) is a life-saving procedure involving removal of large portions of the skull to relieve intracranial pressure in patients with space occupying cerebral edema such as traumatic brain injury (TBI) and stroke. Although the procedure has been shown to decrease mortality in patients, the risk of severe disability is significant. Quality of life, not just survival, following DHC has emerged as an important consideration when the decision is made to perform a DHC.

> With advances in technology, the options to manage patients with neurologic injuries are often complex. Critical care management of neurologic injury has historically focused on the prevention of secondary ischemic injury through aggressive management of intracranial pressure (ICP) and maintenance of adequate cerebral perfusion pressure (CPP). However, ICP monitoring alone does not identify ischemic changes that herald patient deterioration. Advocates of multimodality monitoring cite the value of early detection of changes in brain oxygenation levels and brain metabolism as advantageous in optimizing stroke outcomes. ICP monitoring alone should not be the sole source of information on which therapy is guided but should be incorporated into the arsenal of emerging and promising invasive neuromonitoring devices.

Despite contemporary rehabilitation strategies, stroke remains a leading cause of loss of function, limited mobility, psycho-social complications, and decreased quality of life. Stroke rehabilitation is a process that aims to prevent deterioration of function, increase function, and assist the patient in achieving the highest possible level of independence physically, socially, spiritually, psychologically, vocationally, and economically. The process begins with relearning activities of daily living such as grooming, bathing, toileting, eating, and dressing. As the patient progresses, stroke rehabilitation works on instrumental activities of daily living such as housekeeping, cooking, driving, and managing financial responsibilities.

CRITICAL CARE NURSING
CLINICS OF NORTH AMERICA

SERIES OF RELATED INTEREST

Nursing Clinics of North America http://www.nursing.theclinics.com

---

THE CLINICS ARE AVAILABLE ONLINE!
Access your subscription at:
www.theclinics.com

Preface

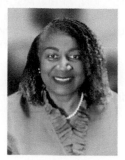

Wandria Dallas, MN, APRN, AGCNS-BC
Editor

A stroke can happen to anyone at any time. Every year, nearly 800,000 Americans suffer a stroke. Despite improvements in stroke treatment in the United States, stroke remains the second leading cause of death worldwide. Stroke is also the third-leading cause of death and disability combined. Worldwide, the annual rate of stroke is 15 million. Of these, 3 million die and another 3 million are left permanently disabled. Stroke occurs every 40 seconds. Rapid and effective evaluation, identification, diagnosis, and treatment of stroke are vital in decreasing stroke morbidity and mortality. Stroke is a disease that is 85% preventable.

Stroke prevention is related to the management of other health conditions and disparities. Age trends, geographic locations, and access to care challenge the professional care of stroke.

The community relies on their health care providers to direct them in matters of their personal health. Nurses and other health care professionals are expected to actively participate in educating their patients and the community to understand stroke and the care provided. Nurses and other health care professionals need to be educated regarding new developments and complex issues in the management of stroke.

This issue of *Critical Care Nursing Clinics of North America* is dedicated nurses and other health care professionals who care for stroke. The topics are designed to increase the understanding of stroke pathophysiology, assist to accurately perform,

Crit Care Nurs Clin N Am 35 (2023) ix–x
https://doi.org/10.1016/j.cnc.2022.12.001
0899-5885/23/© 2022 Published by Elsevier Inc.

ccnursing.theclinics.com

and interpret the assessed needs of stroke, and apply evidence-based practice for improved stroke outcomes.

Wandria Dallas, MN, APRN, AGCNS-BC
Ochsner Louisiana State
University Health Shreveport
1541 Kings Highway
Shreveport, LA 71103, USA

E-mail address:
wandria.dallas@ochsnerlsuhs.org

Strokes and Predictors of Outcomes

Shavonne Williams, MN, APRN, ACNS-BC, ANVP-BC, SCRN, CCRN-K[a],*,
Kimberly Glaser, MSN, APRN, AGACNP-BC, CCRN[b,c], Bappaditya Ray, MBBS, MD[b,d]

KEYWORDS

- Ischemic stroke • Intracerebral hemorrhage • Subarachnoid hemorrhage
- Predictors • Outcomes • Treatment

KEY POINTS

- Stroke is a leading cause of long-term disability.
- Early treatment can improve outcomes in stroke patients.
- Risk versus benefit should be assessed while treating all stroke subtypes.
- Tools to predict outcome are available that vary among different stroke types, and each has its own challenges and requires refinement because new knowledge is gathered and treatment modalities are implemented in the future.

INTRODUCTION

Clinical outcome prediction after a cerebrovascular event is important information for a health-care provider so that he/she can convey that information to the patient, family, close friends, and other health-care providers. Predicting physical disabilities, cognitive outcome, and quality of life after stroke are relevant questions but, unfortunately, without definite answers. Prognosis can affect treatment options that are offered by providers, may affect treatments chosen by the patient and the families, and may directly impact mortality, especially considering the risk for self-fulfilling prophecies associated with clinical practice. The purpose of this review is to examine factors that contribute to prognosis in each stroke subtype.

BACKGROUND

Stroke is a debilitating disease that is due to pathologic condition in brain arteries.[1] It can be due to either blockage of a blood vessel carrying oxygen to the brain (ischemic)

[a] Texas Health Presbyterian Hospital, 8200 Walnut Hill Lane, Dallas, TX 75231, USA; [b] University of Texas Southwestern Medical Center, 5232 Harry Hines, Boulevard MC 8897, Dallas, TX 75039-8897, USA; [c] William P. Clements Jr. University Hospital, 5151 Harry Hines Boulevard, Dallas, TX 75390, USA; [d] Department of Neurology and Neurological Surgery (Neurocritical Care Division), 5323 Harry Hines Boulevard MC 8897, Dallas, TX 75390-8897, USA
* Corresponding author. 3540 East Broad Street, STE 120-226, Mansfield, TX 76063.
E-mail address: leatricewilliams@texashealth.org

Crit Care Nurs Clin N Am 35 (2023) 1–15
https://doi.org/10.1016/j.cnc.2022.10.003
0899-5885/23/© 2022 Elsevier Inc. All rights reserved.

or due to a blood vessel rupture (hemorrhagic).[1] Approximately 87% of strokes are ischemic and about 13% are hemorrhagic.[2] Stroke is a leading cause of long-term disability and accounts for the fifth leading cause of death in the United States annually.[2] Hence, a provider's treatment decision plays an important role in stroke management and outcomes.

ACUTE ISCHEMIC STROKE
Treatment Options for Acute Ischemic Stroke

Principles of acute ischemic stroke (AIS) management involve reestablishing blood flow in blocked cerebral circulation, either through dissolving the clot with systemic or intravenous (IV) recombinant tissue plasminogen activator (rt-PA) or physically removing the clot by means of mechanical thrombectomy (MT). Complications such as symptomatic brain hemorrhage can occur after IV rt-PA but when given within the appropriate time window, patients experienced improved outcomes at 3 months.[3] Tenecteplase (TNK) is another form of IV rt-PA now used for stroke. However, because its clinical use is relatively new, this article will refer to Alteplase, or IV rt-PA, when referencing thrombolytics.

MT can be used in conjunction with thrombolytics or alone. However, because MT is indicated only in treatment of proximal cerebral vessels, thrombolytics still remain the cornerstone of acute stroke therapy.[4] Despite the risks associated with it, patients who undergo MT have favorable outcomes.[5]

Predicting Outcomes in Acute Ischemic Stroke

Prompt medical treatment is important to reduce the impact of long-term disability and mortality in AIS. However, various clinical presentations commonly complicate a provider's decision on how to treat AIS. Over the years, several scoring systems have been developed to guide clinicians in predicting clinical outcomes but none is without drawbacks or widely used (**Table 1** shows some selected scoring systems in AIS). Among these scoring systems, factors such as the modified Rankin Scale (mRS), age, stroke severity and location, diabetes, and stroke volumes contribute across several scores, and we will discuss these in further detail.

Modified Rankin Scale

The mRS reports level of patients' physical functional independence after a stroke. Scores range from 0 (fully independent) to 6 (dead). Several randomized clinical trials have determined mRS to be valid and reliable tool, and thus, mRS is recommended and commonly used as an outcome measure in AIS studies.[13]

A prestroke mRS also help providers to assess preexisting disabilities before acute stroke therapy. Acute treatment may not be beneficial in a patient with a baseline mRS of 5 compared with a patient with a baseline mRS of 0 or 1. Furthermore, patients with preexisting disabilities who undergo acute stroke therapy have increased mortality as well as reduced neurologic improvement.[14] Some of the scoring systems include premorbid mRS as a factor in predicting clinical outcome (see **Table 1**).

Age

Age is a nonmodifiable risk factor for stroke that poses challenges in determining treatment and outcomes because blood vessels in the brain undergo changes with aging as well as brain plasticity to facilitate rehabilitation.[15] Yousufuddin and Young[16] determined about three-quarters of AIS occur in people aged 65 years or older. As more people reach this age, the number of strokes is expected to increase, and older patients with AIS suffer poorer quality of life with higher mortality rates than younger patients.[17]

Table 1
Example of predictive scoring systems for acute ischemic stroke

Totaled Health Risks in Vascular Events[6]		
Factor	Criteria	Score
NIHSS	11–20	2
	≥21	4
Age	60–79 y	1
	≥80 y	2
Hypertension	Yes	1
Diabetes mellitus	Yes	1
Atrial fibrillation	Yes	1
		0–9 (Higher Score is associated with worse outcomes)
Stroke Prognosis Instrument 2 (SPI2)[7,8]		
Congestive heart failure	Yes	3
Diabetes mellitus	Yes	3
Prior stroke	Yes	3
Age >70 y	Yes	2
Stroke (not TIA)	Yes	2
Severe hypertension	Yes	1
Coronary artery disease	Yes	1
	Risk of stroke or death within 2 y after AIS or TIA	0–2 Low-risk group 3–6 Middle-risk group 7–11 High-risk group
GADIS[9]		
Gender	Male	0
	Female	2
Age	<65 y	0
	≥65 y	2
Diabetes mellitus history	Yes	2.5
	No	0
Infarct volume	<17 mL	0
	≥17 mL	4
		<6 points: predicted a mRS of 0–2 at discharge in patients getting MT
iSCORE[10,11]		
Age		+Age (y)
Gender	Male	+10
	Female	0
Stroke severity * measured by using the Canadian Neurologic Scale	0	+105
	≤4	+65
	5–7	+40
	≥8	0
Stroke subtype	Lacunar	0
	Nonlacunar	+30
	Undetermined cause	+35
Risk factor	Atrial fibrillation	+10
	CHF	+10

(continued on next page)

Table 1 (continued)		
Totaled Health Risks in Vascular Events[6]		
Comorbid condition	Cancer	+10
	Renal dialysis	+35
Preadmission disability	Independent	0
	Dependent	+15
Glucose on admission	<135 mg/dL	0
	≥ 135 mg/dL	+15
		<200 points: linked to better outcomes at 3-mo after tPA
PLAN[12]		
Preadmission comorbidities	Cancer	1.5
	Dependence	1.5
	CHF	1
	Atrial fibrillation	1
Level of consciousness	Decreased	5
Age	Per decade	1
		*max 10
Neurologic deficit	Significant or total:	2
	• Leg weakness	2
	• Arm weakness	1
	Neglect or aphasia	1
		Predicted disability and death in patients with AIS Max Score: 25 Score >15 associated with higher mortality rates at 30 d and 1 y >15 associated with higher death or severe disability at discharge

Abbreviation: CHF, Congestive Heart Failure.

Knowing the risks that come with age, some clinicians question whether the prognosis is worth the risk when treating older patients. To provide insight, Bluhmki and colleagues[18] reported that administering IV tPA within the guidelines in patients aged greater than 80 years led to better outcomes than in those who did not get IV tPA. However, an individual risk–benefit assessment was emphasized before administering Alteplase for AIS.[18] In contrast, Martini and colleagues looked at patients aged less than 80 years and those aged 80 years or older who met criteria for MT in anterior circulation strokes and found that postthrombectomy 90-day mRS was higher in older patients.[19]

Although outcomes may vary in older patients after acute stroke intervention, old age alone is not a contradiction to offer such therapy. Older age carries a higher risk of unfavorable outcomes; therefore, risk–benefit should be assessed and shared decision-making with the patient (if possible) and family members is recommended for all before treatment.

Stroke Severity and Location

Stroke severity in AIS is commonly assessed by using the National Institutes of Health Stroke Scale (NIHSS). The NIHSS is regarded as the gold standard for measuring stroke severity and clinicians use it to quickly assess strokes.[20] This 42-point scale focuses on level of consciousness, sensation, neglect, language, and visual, cerebellar, and motor function; higher NIHSS scores represent a greater level of severity.[21] A baseline NIHSS score is a strong and important predictor of functional outcomes, and patients with higher NIHSS admission scores are more likely to have unfavorable outcomes at 90 days.[22–24] In addition to the NIHSS, the extent of completed stroke at presentation also plays a role in outcomes. Patients who present with irreversible injury on computed tomography imaging are likely to have poor prognosis.[14] However, much has changed in the last decade with successful MT trials and reports of large vessel occlusion (both anterior and posterior circulation) with improved clinical outcome in patients with higher preintervention NIHSS and proper selection using advanced neuroimaging studies.

AIS due to basilar artery occlusion (BAO) can be catastrophic, leading to coma and death when left undetected and untreated. Guenego[25] and colleagues explored the benefit of MT in patients with BAO with AIS that were comatose and noncomatose and reported higher mortality and much worse outcomes in comatose patients.[25] Patient outcomes depend on the presence of collateral blood flow to support at risk areas of the brain, early recognition, reperfusion, and if integral parts of the brainstem are affected.[26]

Diabetes Mellitus

Diabetes mellitus increases susceptibility to pathologic changes in blood vessels that can lead to stroke.[27] Hence, diabetes mellitus is a known vascular risk factor for stroke and is reported to be associated with worse outcomes.[28] Furthermore, uncontrolled glucose levels lead to higher mortality with admission hyperglycemia being associated with poorer outcomes.[27,28] Stroke precipitates a stress response that causes systemic hyperglycemia. This hyperglycemia decreases salvageable brain tissue, increases lactate production, and is associated with larger infarct volumes. The phenomenon is highly associated with poorer outcomes.[27] Stress hyperglycemia is associated with poor functional outcomes, however, whether it is a target for intervention that can decrease morbidity is currently unknown. The SHINE trial targeting this phenomenon did not show any difference between control and intervention groups.[29]

Stroke Volume

Malignant cerebral infarction (MCI) is a large volume hemispheric infarct that is associated with life-threatening cerebral edema. MCI carries an 80% mortality rate if not surgically treated. Decompressive hemicraniectomy (DHC), which is surgical removal of part of that skull, prevents fatal cerebral herniation.[30] Early DHC (within 48 hours of stroke) is associated with better neurologic outcomes. DHC leads to improved survival rates, however, only some patients show better functional outcomes with an improvement in quality of life between 1 and 3 years.[31] Hence, it is recommended that post-DHC survival and quality of life be discussed before DHC.[30]

Intracerebral Hemorrhage

Nontraumatic intracerebral hemorrhage (ICH) is the second most common type of stroke in the United States, accounting for about 10% of all stroke, and is due to ruptured intraparenchymal blood vessels.[32,33] Brain damage in ICH occurs from mass effect resulting in cell death and edema from the hematoma breakdown.[33] ICH due to hypertensive cause are commonly located in the basal ganglia, thalamus, brainstem (especially the pons), and cerebellum while ICH due to amyloid angiopathy is most common in the cerebral cortex.[33] Nonmodifiable risk factors for ICH include sex (men are usually more than women), age (older than 40 years is likely hypertensive, older than 60 years is increasingly cerebral amyloid angiopathy), and race (Blacks and Mexican Americans increased risk).[32,34] Apart from primary ICH (ie, any underlying pathologic condition), it can occur due to vascular malformations, cerebral venous thrombosis, sympathomimetic drug use, eclampsia, and brain tumors. Unfortunately, mortality from ICH has been relatively stable during the years at approximately 40% mortality at 30 days.[35] In addition, with increase in elderly population and increased detection of atrial fibrillation with concomitant use of anticoagulants, incidence of ICH has already trebled in the last 25 years and is expected to treble by 2050.[36]

Predicting Outcomes in Intracerebral Hemorrhage

ICH prognosis can be challenging as patients often present in a critical condition situation, confounded with self-fulfilling prophecies and can result in fatal outcome if initial aggressive treatment is not pursued. However, overaggressive treatment approaches and unrealistic family expectations regarding functional recovery can also result in painful interventions, potential patient suffering, waste of essential resources, and adds to health-care burden. Surgical interventions, such as hematoma evacuation to decrease mass effect and prevent fatal cerebral herniation and decompressive craniectomy (ie, removal of cranial bone to allow room for brain swelling, especially in posterior fossa), can be lifesaving. Similarly, when such surgical interventions are not indicated, placement of an extraventricular drain can be inserted to monitor intracranial pressure and maintain optimal cerebral perfusion pressure to prevent secondary brain damage. However, early prognostication can play a crucial factor in determining surgical intervention, especially if patient's clinical condition is determined to be potentially fatal. The following prognostic tools may guide clinicians in predicting outcome.

Intracerebral Hemorrhage Scores

Several scoring systems to assess disease severity and delineate prognosis in ICH are available; however, the ICH score is most commonly used.[32] It is a simple and validated tool that assigns points based on the Glasgow Coma Scale (GCS) at presentation, whether the patient is aged 80 years or older, whether there is presence of intraventricular hemorrhage (IVH), if the location is infratentorial (below the tentorium, where the cerebellum resides), and whether the estimated volume of the ICH hematoma is greater than 30 mL. Higher the score, the higher is the 30-day mortality.[37] Of note, ICH score was developed using a retrospective single center cohort and subsequently validated on a prospective cohort with comparable accuracy.[37] Because this was a single-center study, it is unknown how much local practice pattern might reflect on patient outcome and if ICH score might have real-world validation. Despite the ICH score being the first developed and most known scoring system for ICH, not all neurointensivists use it.[38] Additionally, it has been observed that use of a prognostic score resulted in practice pattern change in management of ICH and, furthermore, that with changes in the practice of medicine today, patient survival surpasses what the original ICH score data predicted.[39,40]

Of note, mortality scores are higher because they include patients who had do not resuscitate (DNR) orders placed early in their care. In fact, continuing full care for at least 5 days resulted in a 30% reduction in mortality.[41] Another scoring tool, the max-ICH score, is similar to the ICH score; however, the researchers sought to improve its accuracy through optimizing severity assessment and accounting for early care withdrawal.[42] The max-ICH score minimizes early care limitations, such as withholding treatments or withdrawal of care, and is likely better in predicting meaningful outcomes for patients who received treatment.[34,43] Elements that comprise the max-ICH score are age, the NIHSS, ICH volume, presence of IVH, and if the patient was taking oral anticoagulants at the time of the bleed.

The FUNC score aimed to address limitations of the other ICH scoring systems and is better at predicting functional recovery.[44] Designed to be useful at the time of admission, it includes the volume of the ICH, age, location of the ICH, the GCS score, and presence of cognitive impairment before the ICH.[44] The FUNC score specifically followed ICH survivors, thus eliminating any mortality interference of early withdrawal of care.[44] It is able to predict patients who are likely to have functional independence at 90 days.[44] In contrast to the other tools, where the higher the score, the poorer the outcome, the FUNC score predicts a better outcome with higher scores. **Table 2** outlines and compares these 3 scoring systems.

Predictor Components

The prediction tools share similar elements, such as age, ICH volume, and GCS score. Each piece of the puzzle affects likelihood of recovery in different ways. Older age, neurologic impairment, antithrombotic/anticoagulant therapy at the time of the bleed, hemorrhage volume, and biomarkers, such as stress hyperglycemia, are the most noteworthy factors.[45]

Age

Age is a well-studied and strong predictor of functional outcome. In fact, older age incrementally associated higher mortality and functional dependency compared with younger patients. Patients aged older than 75 years had a 5 times higher chance of physical disability or death.[46]

Glasgow Coma Scale

Neurologic impairment at the time of admission with an ICH can be used for long-term mortality predictions.[45] Often measured with the GCS, the more severe the neurologic deficit, the worse the predicted outcome. Multiple studies used GCS to grade neurologic deficit, and lower GCS is universally associated with worse clinical outcome.[37,47,48] GCS alone performed just as well as other ICH predictor tools in predicting 30-day mortality.[47]

Antiplatelet and Anticoagulant Therapy

Patients who experience an ICH while on oral anticoagulants are at higher risk of early mortality.[45] When compared with patients who were not on an anticoagulant, patients who took an anticoagulant had higher in-hospital mortality.[49] When compared with patients who took a single antiplatelet therapy against patients taking a combination therapy, those on the combination therapy had higher in-patient mortality.[50] However, although in-hospital mortality was increased, functional outcome of surviving patients was not necessarily poor.[51]

Hemorrhage Volume

The size of the resultant hematoma in an ICH is associated with mortality, with the larger the volume being associated with higher mortality.[45,52] Furthermore, growth of the hematoma in the first day of the bleed also led to worsened mortality and functional outcomes.[53] ICH volume is the single-most image-related factor in mortality prediction.[45]

Table 2
Intracerebral hemorrhage score comparisons

Max-ICH Score		ICH Score		FUNC Score	
Element	Points	Element	Points	Element	Points
Age (y)		Age (y)		Age (y)	
≥80	3	≥80	1	<70	2
75–79	2	<80	0	70–79	1
70–74	1			≥80	0
≤69	0				
NIH Stroke Scale		Glasgow Coma Scale		Glasgow Coma Scale	
≥21	3	3–4	2	≥9	2
14–20	2	5–12	1	≤8	0
7–13	1	13–15	0		
0–6	0				
ICH volume (mL)		ICH volume (mL)		ICH volume (mL)	
Lobar ≥30	1	≥30	1	<30	4
Lobar <30	0	<30	0	30–60	2
Nonlobar ≥10	1			>60	0
Nonlobar <10	0				
Intraventricular hemorrhage		Intraventricular hemorrhage		Pre-ICH cognitive impairment	
Yes	1	Yes	1	No	1
No	0	No	0	Yes	0
Oral anticoagulation		Infratentorial ICH		ICH location	
Yes	1	Yes	1	Lobar	2
No	0	No	0	Deep	1
				Infratentorial	0
Total points	0–9		0–6		0–11

ICH: higher the score, higher the mortality risk.[42]
  Max-ICH: Higher the score, greater chance of decreased functional outcomes.[42]
  FUNC: Higher score is associated with better functional outcomes.[44]

Stress Hyperglycemia

Many patients who have an ICH have hyperglycemia on presentation. Conventionally, blood glucose of 8 mmol/L or greater or 144 mg/dL is considered hyperglycemia. However, recent studies define stress hyperglycemia more individually based on patients' preadmission glycated hemoglobin (HbA1c) and admission serum glucose.[54] However, patients who are persistently hyperglycemic during the first 24 to 72 hours have a worse 6-month mortality. The cause of such increased mortality is unknown but it is speculated that high blood sugars worsen secondary brain injury through potentiating oxidative stress.[55]

Subarachnoid Hemorrhage

Nontraumatic subarachnoid hemorrhage (SAH) is the second most common type of hemorrhagic stroke, which accounts for 2% to 7% of all strokes.[56] Most SAH are due to a ruptured aneurysm, with only about 10% nonaneurysmal perimesencephalic and 5% from other causes.[57] Other causes of SAH include infections, toxins (such as amphetamines, cocaine, and others), blood diseases (such as sickle cell anemia, leukemia, and others), and neoplasms.[57] Although, SAH mortality is decreasing, with about 35% in-hospital mortality, of which 12% to 15% die before making it to the hospital.[57]

Brain injury due to SAH can occur immediately, when an aneurysm ruptures, commonly referred to as early brain injury. It can also occur later in the patient's course as part of a constellation of potential complications and is referred to as delayed cerebral ischemia (DCI).[57] DCI is most common on days 3 through 14 after the initial bleed and is a major factor in delayed neurologic deterioration in SAH.[57] Multiple pathophysiological processes contribute to DCI, including cerebral vasospasm, cortical spreading ischemia, microthromboembolism, and others.[57]

PREDICTING OUTCOMES IN SUBARACHNOID HEMORRHAGE

Most frequently used clinical grading systems to predict clinical outcome are the Hunt and Hess (H&H) grade and the World Federation of Neurological Surgeons (WFNS) scale. The H&H scale describes clinical symptoms of patients and was originally developed to determine surgical risk in aneurysmal SAH, whereas the WFNS scale is designed to be a grading system on clinical aspect of patients who suffered a SAH.[58,59] It is common to see one or both scales mentioned when describing a patient with an SAH. However, these scales do not independently predict functional outcome in patients who experienced SAH but have contributory roles as predictors in scoring systems.

Most patients surviving SAH have cognitive deficits, rather than focal motor deficits, and outcome assessment tools are not sensitive enough to predict meaningful outcomes as compared with ICH.[56] Common deficits include executive dysfunction, impaired short-term memory, concentration problems, fatigue, anxiety, depression, and impulsivity.[56] Multiple tools attempt prognostication and are enumerated in **Table 3**. However, as of this time, none is widely integrated in clinical practice.[56,60-62]

Old age is one of the most notable predictors of poor outcomes in SAH.[63] Approximately 15% to 20% of SAHs occur in patients aged older than 70 years. Long-term disability and mortality rates are higher in older patients with SAH, as opposed to younger patients.[64] The initial hemorrhage as well as recurrent hemorrhage is thought to be the rationale for poorer outcomes in the older population.[65] Additionally, Fehnel and colleagues[64] examined the outcome of older patients treated in facilities with low SAH treatment volume centers and found patient outcome to be better in higher volume centers.

Nursing Assessment and Implications

Several recommendations for stroke management are similar across the different types of strokes. Blood pressure (BP) control goals tend to differ among the different stroke types. Patients who received thrombolytics only for AIS must maintain BP less than 180/105 for 24 hours after treatment.[69] In contrast, ICH guidelines recommend that it is safe for patients who present with systolic BPs (SBP) between 150 and 220 mm Hg to lower BP to 130 to 140 mm Hg.[34] SAH patients should have SBPs lowered to less than 160 mm Hg.[70] Furthermore, to prevent hyperglycemia in AIS, guidelines support maintaining a blood glucose range of 140 to 180 mg/dL and close monitoring to avert hypoglycemia.[14] Cautious management of glucose levels, while preventing hyperglycemia and hypoglycemia, is also important in patients with hemorrhagic stroke.[34,70]

Nurses help affect outcomes by obtaining thorough histories of medications, especially anticoagulants and antiplatelet drugs as reversal of the drugs may be necessary in hemorrhagic strokes. Diligent neurologic examinations in all stroke types may reveal

Table 3
ubarachnoid hemorrhage predictor system examples

CRIG[66]

Clinical/radiological factor	Clinical	128
	Radiological (3–4)	68
	Inflammatory dysGlycemia	1 per unit
		5 per unit
		Score of ≥109 is associated with poor clinical outcomes

SAFIRE[67]

Age	<50y	0
	50–60y	1
	60–70y	2
	≥70y	5
WFNS after resuscitation	1	0
	2	2
	3	3
	4	6
	5	9
Aneurysm size	<10 mm	0
	10–19.9 mm	2
	≥20 mm	6
Fisher grade	1–3	0
	4	2
	Risk of poor outcomes	0–2 Low risk
		3–5 Low-intermediate risk
		6–8 Intermediate risk
		9–15 Intermediate-high risk
		>15 High risk

FRESH[68]

Hunt & Hess		Score on admission
APACHEphys		APACHE physiologic score without GCS
Age	>70	9
	≤70	0
Rebleed in 48 h	Yes	4
	No	0
		The higher the score, the greater the risk of an unfavorable outcome

deterioration. Attentive nurses can prevent medical complications by recognizing swallowing dysfunction, mobility impairments, hemodynamic instability, altered vital signs, including fevers, and signs of delirium. Cognitive and physical rehabilitation from physical, occupational, and speech therapists as soon as medically feasible ensures the best possible return to baseline functioning. Dysphagia, common in stroke patient, can lead to complications such as aspiration pneumonia, dehydration, and malnutrition. Nurse bedside swallow screening should be performed before allowing any oral intake and appropriate referrals should be initiated as needed. These factors complicate hospitalization in addition to increasing mortality and negatively impacting quality of life after stroke.[69]

Nurses should also educate patients and families on the importance of controlling individual risk factors with hopes of minimizing the chances of stroke recurrence as well as offer resources for stroke support groups. The awareness of new physical and cognitive decline can lead to depression in stroke survivors and caregivers. Participation in stroke support groups provides an opportunity for social support, which has been related to better functional outcomes.[71]

Finally, families and medical decision-makers often look to the nurse for feedback on the patient's condition. In the absence of previous delineated documentation by the patient on desires for care, nurses should be aware that patients with full treatment experienced more favorable than anticipated outcomes and, should a patient have a DNR in place, it does not mean do not treat but only do not attempt resuscitation in the event of a cardiopulmonary collapse.

SUMMARY

There are different types of strokes and each has its own specific risks, complications, and concerns. Much research is ongoing into improving treatment options for all strokes, as well as better predicting how much disability a patient may endure. As nurses, we can positively affect stroke patients by recognizing a stroke, administering stroke treatments, assessing for neurologic decline, assisting in therapies, or offering comfort to the patients and their families. Nurses are the caregivers primarily at the bedside, many times experiencing the struggle alongside the patient and family. Awareness of the factors involved in determining patient outcomes can afford the opportunity to recognize issues and potentially pivotally alter the patient's course.

DISCLOSURE

The authors have no conflicts of interest, financial or otherwise.

ACKNOWLEDGMENTS

Samir Shah, MD, Texas Health Presbyterian Hospital Dallas. Chloe D. Villavaso, MN, APRN, ACNS-BC, FPCNA, AACC, Tulane University School of Medicine. Shirley Martin, Ph.D., RN, CPN, Nurse Scientist, Texas Health Presbyterian Hospital Dallas. Viviana Hornick, MLS, Medical Librarian Texas Health Presbyterian Hospital Dallas.

REFERENCES

1. About stroke. American stroke association. Available at: stroke.org/en/about-stroke. Accessed July 20, 2022.
2. Types of stroke and treatment. American stroke association. Available at: https://www.stroke.org/en/about-stroke/types-of-stroke. Accessed August 5, 2022.
3. Group NIoNDaSr-PSS. Tissue plasminogen activator for acute ischemic stroke. N Engl J Med 1995;333(24):1581–7.
4. Mathews S, De Jesus O. Thrombectomy. StatPearls. StatPearls Publishing Copyright © 2022. StatPearls Publishing LLC.; 2022.
5. Rennert RC, Wali AR, Steinberg JA, et al. Epidemiology, natural history, and clinical presentation of large vessel ischemic stroke. Neurosurgery 2019;85(suppl_1):S4–8.
6. Flint AC, Cullen SP, Rao VA, et al. The THRIVE score strongly predicts outcomes in patients treated with the Solitaire device in the SWIFT and STAR trials. Int J Stroke 2014;9(6):698–704.

7. Chaudhary D, Abedi V, Li J, et al. Clinical risk score for predicting recurrence following a cerebral ischemic event. Front Neurol 2019;10:1106.

8. Kernan WN, Viscoli CM, Brass LM, et al. The stroke prognosis instrument II (SPI-II) : a clinical prediction instrument for patients with transient ischemia and non-disabling ischemic stroke. Stroke 2000;31(2):456–62.

9. O'Connor KP, Hathidara MY, Danala G, et al. Predicting clinical outcome after mechanical thrombectomy: the GADIS (gender, age, diabetes mellitus history, infarct volume, and current smoker [corrected]) score. World Neurosurg 2020; 134:e1130–42.

10. Saposnik G, Raptis S, Kapral MK, et al. The iScore predicts poor functional outcomes early after hospitalization for an acute ischemic stroke. Stroke 2011; 42(12):3421–8.

11. Saposnik G, Reeves MJ, Johnston SC, et al. Predicting clinical outcomes after thrombolysis using the iScore: results from the Virtual International Stroke Trials Archive. Stroke 2013;44(10):2755–9.

12. O'Donnell MJ, Fang J, D'Uva C, et al. The PLAN score: a bedside prediction rule for death and severe disability following acute ischemic stroke. Arch Intern Med 2012;172(20):1548–56.

13. Nunn A, Bath PM, Gray LJ. Analysis of the modified Rankin Scale in randomised controlled trials of acute ischaemic stroke: a systematic review. Stroke Res Treat 2016;2016:9482876.

14. Powers WJ, Rabinstein AA, Ackerson T, et al. Guidelines for the early management of patients with acute ischemic stroke: 2019 update to the 2018 guidelines for the early management of acute ischemic stroke: a guideline for healthcare professionals from the American Heart Association/American Stroke Association. Stroke 2019;50(12):e344–418.

15. Bullitt E, Zeng D, Mortamet B, et al. The effects of healthy aging on intracerebral blood vessels visualized by magnetic resonance angiography. Neurobiol Aging 2010;31(2):290–300.

16. Yousufuddin M, Young N. Aging and ischemic stroke. Aging (Albany NY) 2019; 11(9):2542–4.

17. Roy-O'Reilly M, McCullough LD. Age and sex are critical factors in ischemic stroke pathology. Endocrinology 2018;159(8):3120–31.

18. Bluhmki E, Danays T, Biegert G, et al. Alteplase for acute ischemic stroke in patients aged >80 years: pooled analyses of individual patient data. Stroke 2020; 51(8):2322–31.

19. Martini M, Mocco J, Turk A, et al. An international multicenter retrospective study to survey the landscape of thrombectomy in the treatment of anterior circulation acute ischemic stroke: outcomes with respect to age. J Neurointerv Surg 2020; 12(2):115–21.

20. Lyden P. Using the National Institutes of Health stroke scale: a cautionary tale. Stroke 2017;48(2):513–9.

21. Agis D, Goggins MB, Oishi K, et al. Picturing the size and site of stroke with an expanded National Institutes of Health stroke scale. Stroke 2016;47(6):1459–65.

22. Rost NS, Bottle A, Lee JM, et al. Stroke severity is a crucial predictor of outcome: an international prospective validation study. J Am Heart Assoc 2016;5(1):1–7.

23. Wouters A, Nysten C, Thijs V, et al. Prediction of outcome in patients with acute ischemic stroke based on initial severity and improvement in the first 24 h. Front Neurol 2018;9:308.

24. Yao S, Liu X, Luo Y, et al. How strong the predictive ability of the variable age and stroke severity for patients presented late. J Stroke Cerebrovasc Dis 2020;29(2): 104538.
25. Guenego A, Lucas L, Gory B, et al. Thrombectomy for comatose patients with basilar artery occlusion : a multicenter study. Clin Neuroradiol 2021;31(4): 1131–40.
26. Cox M, Kim D, Sedora-Roman NI, et al. Beware the bright basilar artery: an early and specific CT sign of acute basilar artery thrombosis. Intern Emerg Med 2018; 13(8):1327–8.
27. Chen R, Ovbiagele B, Feng W. Diabetes and stroke: epidemiology, pathophysiology, pharmaceuticals and outcomes. Am J Med Sci 2016;351(4):380–6.
28. Lau LH, Lew J, Borschmann K, et al. Prevalence of diabetes and its effects on stroke outcomes: a meta-analysis and literature review. J Diabetes Investig 2019;10(3):780–92.
29. Johnston KC, Bruno A, Pauls Q, et al. Intensive vs standard treatment of hyperglycemia and functional outcome in patients with acute ischemic stroke: the SHINE randomized clinical trial. JAMA 2019;322(4):326–35.
30. Streib CD, Hartman LM, Molyneaux BJ. Early decompressive craniectomy for malignant cerebral infarction: meta-analysis and clinical decision algorithm. Neurol Clin Pract 2016;6(5):433–43.
31. Geurts M, van der Worp HB, Kappelle LJ, et al. Surgical decompression for space-occupying cerebral infarction: outcomes at 3 years in the randomized HAMLET trial. Stroke 2013;44(9):2506–608.
32. Montaño A, Hanley DF, Hemphill JC. Hemorrhagic stroke. Handbook Clin Neurol 2021;176:229–48.
33. Qureshi AI, Mendelow AD, Hanley DF. Intracerebral haemorrhage. Lancet 2009; 373(9675):1632–44.
34. Greenberg SM, Ziai WC, Cordonnier C, et al. Guideline for the management of patients with spontaneous intracerebral hemorrhage: a guideline from the American Heart Association/American Stroke Association. Stroke 2022;53(7): e282–361.
35. van Asch CJJ, Luitse MJA, Rinkel GJE, et al. Incidence, case fatality, and functional outcome of intracerebral haemorrhage over time, according to age, sex, and ethnic origin: a systematic review and meta-analysis. Lancet Neurol 2010; 9(2):167–76.
36. Yiin GS, Howard DP, Paul NL, et al. Age-specific incidence, outcome, cost, and projected future burden of atrial fibrillation-related embolic vascular events: a population-based study. Circulation 2014;130(15):1236–44.
37. Hemphill JC 3rd, Bonovich DC, Besmertis L, et al. The ICH score: a simple, reliable grading scale for intracerebral hemorrhage. Stroke 2001;32(4):891–7.
38. Witsch J, Siegerink B, Nolte CH, et al. Prognostication after intracerebral hemorrhage: a review. Neurol Res Pract 2021;3(1):22.
39. McCracken DJ, Lovasik BP, McCracken CE, et al. The intracerebral hemorrhage score: a self-fulfilling prophecy? Neurosurgery 2019;84(3):741–8.
40. Zahuranec DB, Fagerlin A, Sánchez BN, et al. Variability in physician prognosis and recommendations after intracerebral hemorrhage. Neurology 2016;86(20): 1864–71.
41. Morgenstern LB, Zahuranec DB, Sánchez BN, et al. Full medical support for intracerebral hemorrhage. Neurology 2015;84(17):1739–44.
42. Sembill JA, Gerner ST, Volbers B, et al. Severity assessment in maximally treated ICH patients: the max-ICH score. Neurology 2017;89(5):423–31.

43. Sembill JA, Castello JP, Sprügel MI, et al. Multicenter validation of the max-ICH score in intracerebral hemorrhage. Ann Neurol 2021;89(3):474–84.

44. Rost NS, Smith EE, Chang Y, et al. Prediction of functional outcome in patients with primary intracerebral hemorrhage: the FUNC score. Stroke 2008;39(8):2304–9.

45. Pinho J, Costa AS, Araújo JM, et al. Intracerebral hemorrhage outcome: a comprehensive update. J Neurol Sci 2019;398:54–66.

46. Rådholm K, Arima H, Lindley RI, et al. Older age is a strong predictor for poor outcome in intracerebral haemorrhage: the INTERACT2 study. Age Ageing 2015;44(3):422–7.

47. Parry-Jones AR, Abid KA, Di Napoli M, et al. Accuracy and clinical usefulness of intracerebral hemorrhage grading scores: a direct comparison in a UK population. Stroke 2013;44(7):1840–5.

48. Poon MT, Fonville AF, Al-Shahi Salman R. Long-term prognosis after intracerebral haemorrhage: systematic review and meta-analysis. J Neurol Neurosurg Psychiatry 2014;85(6):660–7.

49. Inohara T, Xian Y, Liang L, et al. Association of intracerebral hemorrhage among patients taking non-vitamin K antagonist vs vitamin K antagonist oral anticoagulants with in-hospital mortality. JAMA 2018;319(5):463–73.

50. Khan NI, Siddiqui FM, Goldstein JN, et al. Association between previous use of antiplatelet therapy and intracerebral hemorrhage outcomes. Stroke 2017;48(7):1810–7.

51. Thompson BB, Béjot Y, Caso V, et al. Prior antiplatelet therapy and outcome following intracerebral hemorrhage: a systematic review. Neurology 2010;75(15):1333–42.

52. Broderick JP, Brott TG, Duldner JE, et al. Volume of intracerebral hemorrhage. A powerful and easy-to-use predictor of 30-day mortality. Stroke 1993;24(7):987–93.

53. Davis SM, Broderick J, Hennerici M, et al. Hematoma growth is a determinant of mortality and poor outcome after intracerebral hemorrhage. Neurology 2006;66(8):1175–81.

54. Li S, Wang Y, Wang W, et al. Stress hyperglycemia is predictive of clinical outcomes in patients with spontaneous intracerebral hemorrhage. BMC Neurol 2022;22(1):236.

55. Wu TY, Putaala J, Sharma G, et al. Persistent hyperglycemia is associated with increased mortality after intracerebral hemorrhage. J Am Heart Assoc 2017;6(8):1–10.

56. Maher M, Schweizer TA, Macdonald RL. Treatment of spontaneous subarachnoid hemorrhage: guidelines and gaps. Stroke 2020;51(4):1326–32.

57. Etminan N, Macdonald RL. Neurovascular disease, diagnosis, and therapy: subarachnoid hemorrhage and cerebral vasospasm. Handb Clin Neurol 2021;176:135–69.

58. WFoNS Committee. Report of world Federation of neurological Surgeons Committee on a universal subarachnoid hemorrhage grading scale. J Neurosurg 1988;68(6):985–6.

59. Hunt WE, Hess RM. Surgical risk as related to time of intervention in the repair of intracranial aneurysms. J Neurosurg 1968;28(1):14–20.

60. Jaja BNR, Saposnik G, Lingsma HF, et al. Development and validation of outcome prediction models for aneurysmal subarachnoid haemorrhage: the SAHIT multinational cohort study. BMJ 2018;360:j5745.

61. Katsuki M, Kakizawa Y, Nishikawa A, et al. Easily created prediction model using deep learning software (Prediction One, Sony Network Communications Inc.) for subarachnoid hemorrhage outcomes from small dataset at admission. Surg Neurol Int 2020;11:374.
62. Witsch J, Kuohn L, Hebert R, et al. Early prognostication of 1-year outcome after subarachnoid hemorrhage: the FRESH score validation. J Stroke Cerebrovasc Dis 2019;28(10):104280.
63. McIntyre MK, Gandhi C, Long A, et al. Age predicts outcomes better than frailty following aneurysmal subarachnoid hemorrhage: a retrospective cohort analysis. Clin Neurol Neurosurg 2019;187:105558.
64. Fehnel CR, Gormley WB, Dasenbrock H, et al. Advanced age and post-acute care outcomes after subarachnoid hemorrhage. J Am Heart Assoc 2017;6(10):1–10.
65. Nieuwkamp DJ, Rinkel GJ, Silva R, et al. Subarachnoid haemorrhage in patients > or = 75 years: clinical course, treatment and outcome. J Neurol Neurosurg Psychiatry 2006;77(8):933–7.
66. Hathidara MY, Campos Y, Chandrashekhar S, et al. Scoring system to predict dospital outcome after subarachnoid hemorrhage-incorporating systemic response: the CRIG score. J Stroke Cerebrovasc Dis 2022;31(8):106577.
67. van Donkelaar CE, Bakker NA, Birks J, et al. Prediction of sutcome after aneurysmal subarachnoid hemorrhage. Stroke 2019;50(4):837–44.
68. Witsch J, Frey HP, Patel S, et al. Prognostication of long-term outcomes after subarachnoid hemorrhage: the FRESH score. Ann Neurol 2016;80(1):46–58.
69. Green TL, McNair ND, Hinkle JL, et al. Care of the patient with acute ischemic stroke (posthyperacute and prehospital discharge): update to 2009 comprehensive nursing care scientific statement: a scientific statement from the American Heart Association. Stroke 2021;52(5):e179–97.
70. Connolly ES Jr, Rabinstein AA, Carhuapoma JR, et al. Guidelines for the management of aneurysmal subarachnoid hemorrhage: a guideline for healthcare professionals from the American Heart Association/American Stroke Association. Stroke 2012;43(6):1711–37.
71. Christensen ER, Golden SL, Gesell SB. Perceived benefits of peer support groups for stroke survivors and caregivers in rural North Carolina. N C Med J 2019;80(3):143–8.

Management of Aspiration Risk in Stroke

Cynthia Cimini, RN, BSN, CCRN, SCRN*, Shawn Moreau, MSN, TCRN, CEN

KEYWORDS

- Pneumonia • Aspiration pneumonia • Stroke • Dysphagia • Aspiration management

KEY POINTS

- Aspiration pneumonia in stroke.
- Stroke complications.
- Dysphagia in stroke.
- Aspiration prevention in stroke.

INTRODUCTION

Stroke-associated pneumonia (SAP) is a major complication in stroke patients and seems to be caused by aspiration.[1] The effects of pneumonia after stroke increase morbidity, mortality, and length of stay (LOS).[1,2] Risk factors for developing SAP are stroke severity, dysphagia, aspiration, mechanical ventilator, and infarct location. Dysphagia is a frequent deficit caused by stroke, occurs up to 78% of the time and is associated with increased aspiration pneumonia.[1] Early recognition of dysphagia with bedside dysphagia screening can assist in preventing the complication of aspiration pneumonia.[3] Screening tools should be evidence based and used within a formal protocol.[2,4] The patient will benefit when a multidisciplinary team plans their care. Physicians, nurses, dieticians, and speech pathologist should communicate to ensure that aspiration prevention strategies are implemented early to optimize patient outcomes.

Incidence of Stroke-Associated Pneumonia

SAP is the recommended term to refer to lower respiratory tract infections within the first 7 days after stroke.[5,6] Reported rates of SAP vary. As many as 50% of patients with stroke in the intensive care unit (ICU) and stroke units and as many as 11% of patients in postacute care rehabilitation experience SAP.[6] Another report indicates SAP incidence as 14% in the first 7 days.[7] It is likely caused by aspiration combined with stroke-induced immunosuppression (SIIS).[1,6] The powerful inflammatory cascade in the brain and the suppression of the peripheral immune system produced by stroke

Rapides Regional Medical Center, 211 Fourth Street, Alexandria, LA 71301, USA
* Corresponding author.
E-mail address: nurcyncim@aol.com

ccnursing.theclinics.com

is called SIIS. The direct clinical consequence of SIIS in stroke patients is an increased susceptibility to infections, which is enhanced by clinical factors such as dysphagia.[8] Aspiration is defined as breathing in or misdirection of a foreign object such as oropharyngeal secretions, gastric contents (emesis), foods or liquids into the larynx and lower respiratory tract. Many times, this happens when protective reflexes are reduced or jeopardized. The infection that can result after this is aspiration pneumonia.[9,10]

Morbidity and Mortality of Pneumonia in Stroke

Poststroke pneumonia is associated with increased morbidity, mortality, and LOS.[1,2] When compared with poststroke survivors whose recovery is not complicated by pneumonia, there is a 3-fold increase in the risk of dying when diagnosed with pneumonia after stroke.[11] The mortality rate in patients who develop pneumonia is 21% versus 4.8% in those without pneumonia. LOS is also increased in those who develop pneumonia and have a median of 14 days versus 5 days in those who do not develop pneumonia.[2] Increase in morbidity and LOS have shown to increase medical cost as well.[3,4,9,11]

Factors that Affect a Stroke Patient's Risk for Pneumonia

Factors that affect a stroke patient's risk for SAP are higher stroke severity, dysphagia and aspiration, mechanical ventilation, brain stem infarction, large middle cerebral artery (MCA) infarction, and left anterior cerebral artery infarction.[6] Pneumonia caused by aspiration is connected to a high prevalence of dysphagia and in turn it is considered a significant risk factor for pneumonia after stroke.[3,12,13] Risk of pneumonia is 3 times higher in patients with dysphagia.[10]

Dysphagia

Dysphagia is defined as difficulty in swallowing. There are many nerves and muscles in the mouth, cheek, tongue, and pharynx that make swallowing a complex process. Each nerve, structure, and muscle must play its part for the coordinated effort of swallowing and the slightest malfunction in any of these can cause dysphagia. The swallowing process is divided into phases:

First stage: Oral phase—tongue and jaw work together to get food into the consistency needed to swallow.

Second stage: Pharyngeal phase—tongue pushes food or liquid to the back of the mouth and triggers the swallowing response that passes the food through the pharynx. The larynx closes tightly and breathing stops to prevent food or liquid from entering the airway or lungs.

Third stage: Esophageal phase—begins when food enters the esophagus and food is carried to the stomach.[14]

The following cranial nerves that originate in portions of the medulla and pons assist in swallowing with their sensory and motor control[6]:

Medulla

Hypoglossal (CN XII) motor function allows control of the tongue muscles.[6]

Glossopharyngeal (CN IX) motor and sensory function that elevates the palate, controls movement of the pharynx and larynx, and contributes to swallowing through control of the stylopharyngeus muscle; controls sensation from the palate and tongue and taste from the posterior tongue and pharynx.[6]

Vagus (CNX) motor and sensory function controls the muscles and receives sensory input from the pharynx and larynx.[6]

Portions of the accessory nerve (CN XI) motor function innervates the muscle of the larynx, pharynx, trapezius, and sternocleidomastoid muscle.[6]

Pons

Facial (CNVII) motor and sensory function innervates facial muscles and provides parasympathetic supply of the submandibular and sublingual glands providing taste and sensation for the anterior two-thirds of the tongue, hard palate, and soft palate.[6]

Trigeminal (CN V) motor and sensory, which communicates pain, temperature, and light touch from the face and scalp and from the sinuses and oral cavities. The motor fiber innervates the muscle of mastication.[6]

Location of Lesion in Relation to Dysphagia

Dysphagia can occur with unilateral stroke, either right or left, with a slight predominance of the right-sided lesions. There is association in location of ischemic stroke and degree of dysphagia as patients with total middle cerebral artery, brainstem infarction, and capsular infarctions had a high degree of dysphagia. Lesions in the frontoparietal operculum, parietal, parietooccipital, and thalamus, as well, had a high frequent association with dysphagia. In ICH, intraventricular extension was the most common site associated with dysphagia.[15]

Incidence and Risk Factors of Dysphagia After Stroke

Dysphagia is a common complication of stroke, occurring 37% to 78% of patients and is associated with increased aspiration pneumonia, mortality, and poor functional outcomes.[16] A literature review determined the incidence of reported dysphagia after stroke by screening (37%–45%), clinical testing (51%–55%), and instrumental testing (64%–78%). Differences were attributed to variations in method of identification, times of identification after stroke, and lesion location.[13] Khedr discovered dysphagia was found in a higher mean age group for both ischemic and hemorrhagic strokes.[15] Stroke severity and lesion size significantly correlate with the severity of dysphagia in both ischemic and hemorrhagic strokes, as well.[15] Diabetes, hypertension, and atrial fibrillation are associated with dysphagia in the ischemic group.[15] Joundi found that patients that fail dysphagia screening likely:

- Have had a prior stroke,
- Have dementia,
- More often come from a long-term care facility,
- More often present with weakness and speech deficits,
- Have a lower level of consciousness, and
- Have a higher stroke severity,[17]

Dysphagia Screening

The early diagnosis and treatment of dysphagia in stroke patients are important to prevent the development of SAP as well as malnutrition and dehydration.[3,10] It is difficult to determine which patients may have dysphagia when admitted with stroke symptoms without screening.[18] The most important consideration for these patients, initially, is aspiration risk and the suitability for oral feeding.[19] There is a direct benefit of dysphagia screening following acute stroke when screening is administered by trained screeners soon after hospital admission to decrease pneumonia, mortality, dependency, and LOS.[20] Comparison of rates of pneumonia between sites with a formal dysphagia screen protocol was 2.4% versus 5.4% at sites with no formalized screen.[2,21] Palli found that trained nurses can effectively perform a formal bedside dysphagia screen timely 24/7 when speech-language therapists are not initially available.[22] Timely detection of dysphagia fosters prophylactic strategies against aspiration such as nothing by mouth (NPO) status and nasogastric (NG) tube feeding.[22] Failures to recognize dysphagia can also lead to dehydration, malnutrition, and weight loss. Consultation of the dietician to provide the team with patient-specific nutritional needs is necessary.[7] All of these complications can be detrimental to patient outcomes.

Dysphagia (swallow) screen is a pass/fail procedure or tool, which is not diagnostic and is done by a trained nurse to determine whether the patient can eat or drink safely before the speech-language pathologist performs a formal dysphagia assessment.[7] Although dysphagia screening by nurses does not replace assessment by other health professionals, it enhances the provision of care to at-risk patients by allowing early recognition and intervention.[10] The most recent stroke clinical practice guidelines support dysphagia screening to be completed early, preferably on admission, and before oral intake as a Class I recommendation.[7,21,23]

The clinical effectiveness of a dysphagia screening strategy will depend not only on the accuracy and reliability of the screening method but also on the effectiveness of the dysphagia management interventions that follow. There is absence of consensus for a single best swallow screening method; however, swallow screening should still be performed.[24]

A swallow screening procedure should[4]

1. Be valid and reliable,
2. Be quick and minimally invasive,
3. Determine the likelihood of dysphagia and aspiration,
4. Determine whether the patient needs further swallowing assessment, and
5. Determine whether it is safe to feed the patient orally.

There are multiple different dysphagia screening tools available, such as the tools compared in **Table 1**. Stroke care team leaders should work together to select an appropriate one for their facility.

Dysphagia screening should be completed before oral intake, including food, beverages, and oral medication is initiated. The patient will need to be placed NPO until completed. It should be performed by a trained nurse, speech-language pathologist, or other trained health-care provider. Patients who fail screening should be kept NPO and referred to a speech-language pathologist for a full instrumental evaluation swallowing function.[6,7,16] An integrated team approach, clinical pathway, and formal written screening protocol also improve rates of pneumonia. Delays in Speech Licensed Pathologist assessment were associated with SAP with an absolute risk of pneumonia incidence of 1% per day of delay.[21,27] Nurses and speech pathology should keep communication open for the best approach to discover if dysphagia is a problem for the stroke patient.

Other methods of dysphagia evaluation after bedside screening are video fluoroscopy (video swallow), fiber optic, endoscopic evaluation, and comprehensive speech pathology.[6]

Barriers to Completing and Documenting Dysphagia Screening

Compliance in completing dysphagia screening for stroke admissions is a challenge for many facilities. This is apparent in conversations with other stroke coordinators as auditing of compliance is ongoing in these facilities. A Joint Commission standard for stroke centers is that *all* patients with stroke symptoms are screened for dysphagia before oral intake of food, liquid, or medications. I interviewed 5 nurses at 3 different

Table 1
Comparison of a selection of dysphagia screening tool

Test	Components of Test	Strengths	Limitations
Toronto Bedside Swallowing Screening Test (TOR-BSST)[25]	Four items, each assigned a "pass/fail" response (voice before, tongue movements, water swallow, and voice after)	Reliable, sensitive, validated against instrumental assessment	Time (4-h training, 10 min to administer test); proprietary; small sample size in studies
Gugging Swallowing Screen (GUSS)[25,26]	Consists of four subtests (indirect assessment, direct assessment of: swallowing semisolid, liquid, and solid)	Sensitive, single swallowing item; quick and reliable	Studies did not evaluate the screen's capability of preventing aspiration pneumonia
Barnes-Jewish Hospital Stroke Dysphagia Screen[25]	Four items of indirect assessment (LOC, face, tongue, and palate symmetry) and one item of direct swallowing assessment	Sensitive, easy to administer	No recommendations for nutrition/dietary plan

stroke facilities. My findings after interview revealed that all 3 stroke facilities indicated the following barriers for completing and documentation:

1. Many times, the bedside dysphagia screen is completed by the nurse but is documented 1 to 2 minutes after medication administration documentation. Failure to edit the "real time" documentation is apparent because when nurses are confronted as to the sequence of interventions, the response is that they completed the dysphagia screen before medication administration but failed to edit the time.
2. Patients that are intubated on arrival or shortly after may have medications administrated by the NG tube route but the actual medication documentation route is per oral (PO). This indicates per documentation that the medication is given PO but in reality, it is given per NG. Medication routes should be changed. Another scenario for intubated patients is that the nurse forgets to complete and or document screening after extubation.
3. Subtle or mild stroke symptoms prevent the recognition of need for bedside dysphagia screening.
4. Nurses do not understand the implications or effects of dysphagia on patients and that those with even mild stroke symptoms can have detrimental outcomes when this deficit is missed.

Joundi discovered that one in 5 eligible patients with acute ischemic stroke does not receive documented dysphagia screening.[17] Patients with mild strokes often have no documented screening despite the moderate rate of failure and significant risk of complications after failing.[17] It was found that over one-third of patients with mild strokes failed if tested.[17] Failing a dysphagia screening test is a strong and independent predictor of pneumonia, disability, and death.[17] This highlights the importance of dysphagia screening for all patients with acute ischemic stroke.[17] This importance should be relayed to nursing staff on new hire orientation as well as annually to ensure compliance and best outcomes for stroke patients.

Facility Dysphagia Screen Performance Improvement

The American Heart Association Get with the Guidelines (GWTG) - Stroke Plus Measure for annual award recognition is that at least 75% patients undergo screening for dysphagia with bedside testing before being given food, fluids, or medication by mouth. Our facility's 2019 GWTG dysphagia screen measure compliance was 85.9%. The facility stroke team aimed to improve compliance despite meeting the 75% goal for Plus Measure award recognition. An internal process improvement goal of 94% compliance was established to ensure aspiration pneumonia in stroke patients would be at a minimum.

The task force reviewed the process that was already in place, using the Barnes Jewish Tool, to ensure the dysphagia screen was completed in a timely fashion. Educational posters, displayed in the Emergency Department medication rooms, remind the nurses to perform the screen. A reminder was attached to PO aspirin, when administered in the Emergency Department, with the following, "Stroke Symptoms? If so, a bedside swallow study is required before administering PO medication." The tool steps were reviewed as well as the dysphagia screening protocol. The protocol that all new hire nurses were exposed to, as well as annual competency validation education was as follows:

1. Complete and document a dysphagia screen (pass/fail) on all patients with any neurologic symptom before any liquid, food, or oral medication.
2. If the screen is passed, the physician is notified, and a diet is ordered.
3. If the screen is failed, the patient remains NPO until speech therapy (ST) completes an assessment with formalized screening and recommendations.

The inpatient stroke order set includes an ST order for evaluation and treatment. All stroke patients are to be seen by ST within 12 to 24 hours of receiving the consult order. All patients are evaluated regardless of whether the screening is passed or failed.

In Q1 2020 auditing of all stroke patients with a primary diagnosis of stroke for compliance in bedside dysphagia screening began. Nursing unit managers completed one-on-one education to nursing staff that had omitted completing a bedside dysphagia screen before food, fluids, or medications. In Q1 2021, Quality nurses began concurrent chart review of patients admitted with the diagnosis of stroke or documented stroke symptoms on admission for bedside dysphagia screen compliance. Staff nurses were contacted in real time with a reminder to complete if documentation was not found. In Q2 2021, a nursing order for bedside dysphagia screening was added to any Emergency Department Chief Complaint in which symptomology was suspicious of stroke. This order allowed the nurse to have a reminder, in "red," of the need for the dysphagia screen to be completed on the status board or their electronic "to do" list. Data indicating compliance are presented to staff, by individual unit, to encourage staff to continue to strive for excellence, as well as create health competition.

In Q4 2021, our compliance increased to 98.1% from 85.9% in 2019 (**Fig. 1**). Additionally, maintenance of aspiration pneumonia in patients with ischemic stroke has maintained range from 1.3% to 2.9%, well within the established goal.

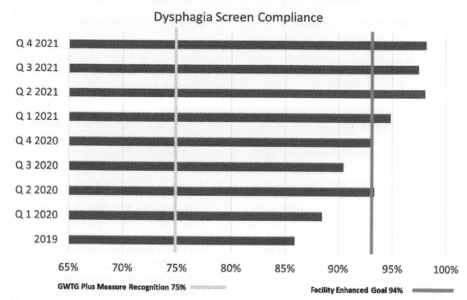

Fig. 1. Dysphagia screening compliance increased from 85.9% in 2019 to 98.1% in 2021.

Nursing Approach for Aspiration Pneumonia Prevention

It is important that nurses complete frequent and ongoing assessments of the patient with stroke to discover any symptom that may allow the detection of dysphagia and their aspiration risk. The features most predictive of aspiration risk include a wet voice, weak voluntary cough, cough on swallowing, prolonged swallow, or combination of these. Bedside swallow tests are safe, therefore can be repeated, and straightforward to perform. Nurses should also understand that many swallow test methods miss silent aspiration.[19] Small–volume aspirations that produce no overt symptoms are common and are often not discovered until the condition progresses to aspiration pneumonia.[10] Patients should be rescreened during the course of the admission as needed or if swallowing or neurologic status changes.[7] This is especially true for patients that have been extubated. These patients should be screened after extubation and before PO intake.[7] Frequent assessments and auscultation of lungs to watch for signs and symptoms of aspiration is important. This would include assessing immediately after feeding or giving liquids. Prompt notification to the physician of any abnormalities to determine treatment modalities is necessary. Signs and symptoms of concern would include the following:

- Audible: A voice change such as hoarseness or a gurgling noise after swallowing.[10]
- Respiratory: dyspnea, tachycardia, cough, wet vocal quality, wheeze, rales, rhonchi, hypoxia, abnormal chest radiograph.[6,9]
- Systemic: Fever, delirium, or confusion, poor feeding, decline in functional status.[6]

Nursing Care of the Patient with Dysphagia

The nurse may institute swallow safety interventions per ST recommendations and aspiration prevention strategies (**Table 2**).

Table 2
Nursing swallow safety and aspiration prevention interventions with rationales

Intervention	Rationale
Administer poststroke aspirin therapy rectally or intravenously if the patient fails the swallow screen[7]	Administration of aspirin is recommended as a Class 1 Level of Evidence in patients with acute ischemic stroke within 24 to 48 h after onset as per clinical practice guidelines[23]
Provide oral feeding only when awake and alert[6,a]	Alertness effects cough reflex and sedation will suppress cough reflex
Provide 30 min rest period before feeding[10]	A rested patient will likely have less difficulty swallowing
Supervise feeding and give frequent cues to swallow with inspection of oral cavity to observe for pocketing of food on one side of the mouth[6,7,a]	Helps identify abnormalities early and allows implementation of strategies for safe swallowing. Withhold fluids and foods as needed to prevent aspiration
Sit patient up in chair or elevate head of bed with oral feeding and maintain for at least 30 min after feeding[6,7,9,10,a]	Keeping patient's head elevated helps keep food in stomach and decreases incidence of aspiration
Flex head to neutral position, chin tuck or head rotation with swallow, depending on type of swallow disorder. For example, a chin down posture is helpful for patients with a tongue base swallowing disorder[6,7,10,a]	Positioning assist with swallowing function by adjusting the anatomy of the throat. These interventions are done at the direction of the speech pathologist
Avoid rushed or forced feeding; adjust rate of feeding to the patient's tolerance[6,10,a]	Well-masticated food is easier to swallow
Provide thickened liquid or a pureed diet[6,7,10,a]	There is easier control of food and liquids, thus preventing premature spillage into the pharynx. Determine the best viscosity with help from speech therapist
Alternate solid and liquid boluses with multiple swallows[7,a]	Liquid and multiple swallows will ensure solid food is safely swallowed
Place medication and food on the strong side of the mouth when unilateral weakness or paresis is present[9]	Careful food placement promotes chewing and successful swallowing
For patients with reduced cognitive abilities, eliminate distracting stimuli during mealtimes. Avoid talking until all food and liquid is swallowed[7,9,a]	Concentration must be focused on chewing and swallowing. There is a higher risk for airway to be opened when talking and eating at the same time
Assess for presence of nausea and vomiting. Antiemetics may be required to prevent aspiration of emesis[7,9]	Vomiting places patients at great risk for aspiration, especially if the level of consciousness is compromised
Auscultate bowel sounds to asses for gastrointestinal motility and observe for abdominal distention[9]	Abdominal distention can be associated with paralytic or mechanical obstruction. Reduced gastrointestinal motility increases the risk of aspiration as fluids and food build up in the stomach. Further, elderly patients have a decrease in esophageal motility, which delays esophageal emptying. When combined with the weaker gag reflex of older patients, aspiration is at higher risk

(continued on next page)

Table 2 (continued)	
Intervention	**Rationale**
Provide frequent oral care including before and after meals[6-7,9,a]	Oral care before meals reduce bacterial counts in the oral cavity. Oral care after eating removes residual food that could be aspirated at a later time

[a] Indicates evidence-based interventions.

Oral care for aspiration pneumonia prevention

Perry recognized the presence of respiratory pathogens in the mouths of acute stroke patients within 48 hours of a stroke and the increased risk of colonization from the respiratory pathogens remained throughout their recovery.[28] These pathogenic organisms could be aspirated and lead to aspiration pneumonia.[10] A Cochrane review that included 3 studies found that oral care and decontamination gel versus oral care and placebo gel reduced the incidence of pneumonia in the intervention group.[23] A study, conducted by Wagner, compared rates of pneumonia in hospitalized stroke patients before and after implementation of systemic oral hygiene care reduced hospital-acquired pneumonia from 14% to 10.33%.[29] Another study indicated intensive oral hygiene protocols using antibacterial mouth rinse with chlorhexidine may reduce SAP from 28% to 7%.[7]

Good oral hygiene is important to minimize the risk of aspiration pneumonia. Missing teeth and poorly fitted dentures predispose to aspiration by interfering with chewing and swallowing. Infected teeth can potentiate the aspiration of contaminated oral secretions.[10] Oral care should be provided frequently to both patients who are eating and those who are NPO as well as patients with tracheostomy or intubation. Brush teeth twice a day and swab mouth with sponge applicators every 2 to 4 hours between brushing if the patient has an artificial airway. An electric suction apparatus should be available during oral care and used any time there is a buildup of oral secretions to prevent aspiration of the oral content.[9] Nursing staff should be provided oral care training. Brady determined that improving staff knowledge also improved their attitude of oral care, which resulted in improved oral hygiene.[30]

Aspiration Prevention During Tube Feeding

Nurses should first feed patients with swallowing difficulty with an NG tube in the early phase of stroke. For those with longer anticipated persistent swallowing difficulty, insertion of a percutaneous gastrostomy (PEG) tube may be warranted. Consult dietician for tube feeding recommendations.[7] PEG feeding is reserved for stroke patients who have persisting dysphagia at 2 to 3 weeks after the stroke. The removal of the feeding tube may be possible for some stroke patients due to spontaneous and or treatment-induced recovery.[10] For most patients, swallowing function returns in 7 days but 11% to 50% may continue having dysphagia 6 months after stroke.[7]

Frequent nursing assessments and safety interventions are needed with tube feeding patients to assist in preventing aspiration (**Table 3**).

Enteral feedings by an NG tube or a PEG tube offers no significant protection against aspiration pneumonia because there is no difference in incidence.[7,10] It is the most common cause of death in PEG-fed patients.[10]

Table 3
Nursing interventions and rationales for patients receiving tube feeding

Intervention	Rationale
Check tube placement before feeding (markings, radiograph, pH of gastric fluid, color of aspirate)[9]	A displaced tube may deliver tube feeding into the airway. Chest radiograph verification of tube placement is most reliable. Gastric aspirate is usually green, brown, clear or colorless, with a pH between 1 and 5.
Monitor tube location every 4 h or per institutional policy[10]	A feeding tube inadvertently displaced into the esophagus greatly increases aspiration risk
Observe for signs of intolerance to feedings such as abdominal distention and large gastric residual volume. Check residuals before feeding or every 4 h, if continuous feeding. Hold feedings if residual is large and notify the physician[9,10]	Patients may not be able to communicate discomfort of distention caused by delayed gastric emptying. If patient is able to communicate, educate patient to notify staff concerning nausea, feeling full, abdominal pain, or cramping. Delayed gastric emptying can lead to reflux and emesis. The amount of residual may vary depending on the volume and rate of infusion. Feedings are often held if residual volume is greater than 50% of the amount delivered in 1 h. Follow intuitional policy or physicians order concerning residuals
Keep head of bed elevated at least 30° during continuous feeding. For intermittent feedings, keep head of bed elevated at least 30° during feedings and for at least an hour afterward[10]	Keeping patient's head elevated helps keep food in stomach and decreases gastric reflux
Stop continual feeding temporarily when turning or positioning patient[9]	When turning or positioning, it is difficult to keep head of bed elevated to prevent gastric reflux
Per physician's order, put several drops of blue or green food coloring in tube feeding to help indicate aspiration. Test glucose in tracheobronchial secretions to detect aspiration of enteral feedings[9]	Colored secretions suctioned or coughed would indicate aspiration

Patient and Family Education

Nurses should begin to educate patients and their families about dysphagia management when diagnosed. Careful explanation of what is being done and why can help reduce fear and anxiety, enhance cooperation and success for patients and their families. The family may try to give liquids or even food when the nurse is not in the room simply because they do not understand the reasoning behind not allowing mother to have a sip when her throat is dry. Food and feeding habits may be strongly tied to family cultural values. Acknowledgment and/or adjustment to cultural values can facilitate compliance and successful family coping. The patient and family should be assessed for willingness and cognitive ability to learn and cope with swallowing disorders.[9] The patient and caregiver should be trained concerning dysphagia management and aspiration prevention. The nurse, dietician, and the speech pathologist can work cooperatively with this endeavor.[7]

SUMMARY

With stroke being the fifth leading cause of death and a leading cause of disability, there is a need for nurses to lead the campaign to reduce stroke complications as much as possible. SAP caused by aspiration and dysphagia is one complication in which nurses can have influence. Because of the increased mortality, morbidity, and the impact on the quality of life, dysphagia needs to be discovered early after the stroke patient's arrival. Nurses are the first line of defense in the patient's battle against aspiration. Early screening to discover dysphagia will set the paradigm in motion for the interdisciplinary team to give the stroke patient the best outcome possible. It is difficult to predict which patients may have dysphagia and be at risk for aspiration without initial screening and ongoing assessments. Most stroke patients have one or more risk factors for dysphagia after stroke, which makes them even more susceptible to aspiration and unfavorable outcomes. Staff education, frequent patient assessment, prevention interventions, and patient/family education is necessary to prevent the complications of aspiration. Gathering data concerning dysphagia screening compliance and identification of opportunities for improvement are instrumental in making change to benefit stroke patients and reduce complications caused by dysphagia and aspiration.

CLINICS CARE POINTS

- Dysphagia is a common complication of stroke, occurs in up to 78% of stroke patients, and is associated with increased aspiration pneumonia, increased mortality, and poor functional outcome.[7,23]
- Diagnosis and treatment of dysphagia with dysphagia screening should be completed early, preferably on admission, and before oral intake.[7,21,23]
- A swallow screen should:
  - Be valid and reliable,
  - Be quick,
  - Be minimally invasive,
  - Determine the likelihood of dysphagia and aspiration,
  - Determine if the patient needs further swallow assessment, and
  - Determine if it is safe to feed the patient.[4,6]
- A team approach, clinical pathway, and formal written screening protocol improve rates of pneumonia.[7,21,23]
- The nurse should institute evidence-based swallow safety strategies for the dysphagia patient to assist with aspiration prevention. See **Table 2**.[6,7]
- The patient and caregiver should be educated about dysphagia, dysphagia management, and aspiration prevention.[7]

DISCLOSURE

The authors have nothing to disclose.

DISCLAIMER

This research was supported (in whole or in part) by HCA Healthcare and/or an HCA Healthcare-affiliated entity. The views expressed in this publication represent those of the authors and do not necessarily represent the official views of HCA Healthcare or any of its affiliated entities.

ACKNOWLEDGMENTS

The authors thank Christy M Seidel, Ph.D., CCC-SLP for her assistance in literature search and guidance for this article. They also thank Shannon Kuczynski, MSN, MHSA, RN, NE-BC for her thoughtful review of this article.

REFERENCES

1. Hannawi Y, Hannawi B, Venkatasubba Rao CP, et al. Stroke-associate pneumonia: major advances and obstacles. Cerebrovasc Dis 2013;35(5):430–43.
2. Hinchey JA, Shephard T, Furie K, et al. Formal dysphagia screening protocols prevent pneumonia. Stroke 2005;36(9):1972–6.
3. Chang MC, Choo YJ, Seo KC, et al. The relationship between dysphagia and pneumonia in acute stroke patients: a systematic review and meta-analysis. Front Neurol 2022;13:834240.
4. Donovan NJ, Daniels SK, Edmiaston J, et al. On behalf of the American Heart association Council on Cardiovascular nursing and stroke Council. Dysphagia screening: state of the art: invitational conference proceeding from the State-of-the-Art nursing Symposium, International stroke Conference 2012. Stroke 2013;44(4):e24–31.
5. Smith CJ, Kishore AK, Vail A, et al. Diagnosis of stroke-associated pneumonia: recommendations from the pneumonia in stroke consensus group. Stroke 2015;46(8):2335–40.
6. Keigher KM, Livesay SL, Wessol JL, editors. Comprehensive review for stroke nursing. 2nd ed. AANN; 2020.
7. Green TL, McNair ND, Hinkle JL, et al. On behalf of the American Heart Association Stroke Nursing Committee of the Council on Cardiovascular and Stroke Nursing and the Stroke Council. Care of the patient with acute ischemic stroke (posthyperacute and prehospital discharge): update to 2009 comprehensive nursing care scientific statement: a scientific statement from the American Heart Association. Stroke 2021;52(5):e179–97.
8. Faura J, Bustamante A, Miro-Mur F, et al. Stroke-induced immunosuppression: implications for the prevention and prediction of post-stroke infections. J Neuroinflammation 2021;18(1):127.
9. Wayne G. Risk for aspiration nursing care plan. Labs risk for aspiration nursing care plan. Nurselabs.com. 2022. Available at: Nurselabs.com/risk-for-aspiration/. Accessed August 1, 2022.
10. Metheny N. Preventing aspiration in older adults with dysphagia. Hign.org. Available at: Hign.org/consultgeri/try-this-series/preventing-aspiration-older-adults-dysphagia. Accessed August 25, 2022.
11. Katzan IL, Cebul RD, Husak BA, et al. The effects of pneumonia on mortality among patients hospitalized for acute stroke. Neurology 2003;60(4):620–5.
12. Lo WL, Leu HB, Yang MC, et al. Dysphagia and risk of aspiration pneumonia: a nonrandomized, pair-matched cohort study. J Dental Sci 2019;14(3):241–7.
13. Martino R, Foley N, Bhogal S, Diamant N, et al. Dysphagia after stroke: incidence, diagnosis, and pulmonary complications. Stroke 2005;36(12):2756–63.
14. Dysphagia: NIDCD fact sheet: voice, speech and language. Nidcd.nih.gov. 2014. Available at: http://www.nidcd.nih.gov/sites/default/files/documenta/health/voice/NIDCD-Dysphagia.pdf. Accessed August 3, 2022.

15. Khedr EM, Abbass MA, Soliman RK, et al. Post-stroke dysphagia: frequency, risk factors, and topographic representation: hospital-based study. Egypt J Neurol Psychiatry Neurosurg 2021;57(23):1–8.
16. Powers WJ, Rabinstein AA, Ackerson T, et al. On behalf of the American Heart Association Stroke Council. Guidelines for the early management of patients with acute ischemic stroke: a guideline for healthcare professionals from the American Heart Association/American Stroke Association. Stroke 2018;49(3): e46–99.
17. Joundi RA, Martino R, Sapsonik G, et al. Predictors and outcomes of dysphagia screening after acute ischemic stroke. Stroke 2017;48(4):900–6.
18. Daniels SK, Pathak S, Mukhi SV, et al. The relationship between lesion localization and dysphagia in acute stroke. Dysphagia 2017;32(6):777–84.
19. Ramsey DJC, Smithard DG, Kalra L. Early assessments of dysphagia and aspiration risk in acute stroke patients. Stroke 2003;34(5):1252–7.
20. Sherman V, Greco E, Martino R. The benefit of dysphagia screening in adult patients with stroke: a meta-analysis. J Am Heart Assoc 2021;10(12):e018753.
21. Greenberg SM, Ziai WC, Cordonnier C, et al. On behalf of the American Heart association/American stroke association. 2022 guideline for the management of patients with spontaneous intracerebral hemorrhage: a guideline from the American Heart association/American stroke association. Stroke 2022;53(7). 2282-e361.
22. Palli C, Fandler S, Doppelhofer K, et al. Early dysphagia screening by trained nurses reduces pneumonia rate in stroke patients. Stroke 2017;48(9):2583–5.
23. Powers WJ, Rabinstein AA, Ackerson T, et al. On behalf of the American Heart Association Stroke Council. Guidelines for the early management of patients with acute ischemic stroke: 2019 update to the 2018 guidelines for the early management of acute ischemic stroke: a guideline for healthcare professionals from the American Heart Association/American Stroke Association. Stroke 2019; 50(12):e344–418.
24. Smith EE, Kent DM, Bulsara KR, et al. Effect of dysphagia screening strategies on clinical outcomes after stroke: a systematic review for the 2018 guidelines for the early management of patients with acute ischemic stroke. Stroke 2018;49(3): e123–8.
25. Oliveira IJ, Mota L, Freitas SV, et al. Dysphagia screening tools for acute stroke patients available for nurses: a systematic review. Nurs Pract Today 2019;6(3): 103–15.
26. Trapl M, Enderle P, Nowotny M, et al. Dysphagia bedside screening for acute-stroke patients. Stroke 2007;38(11):2948–52.
27. Eltringham SA, Kilner K, Gee M, et al. 2018 Impact Of dysphagia assessment and management on risk of stroke-associated pneumonia: a systematic review. Cerebrovasc Dis 2018;46(3):97–105.
28. Perry SE, Jukabee ML, Tompkins G, et al. The association between oral bacteria, the cough reflex and pneumonia in patients with acute stroke and suspected dysphagia. J Oral Rehabil 2019;47(3):386–94.
29. Wagner C, Marchina S, Deveau JA, et al. Risk of stroke associated pneumonia and oral hygiene. Cerebrovasc Dis 2016;41(1–2):35–9.
30. Brady MC, Furlanetto D, Hunter R, et al. Staff-led interventions for improving oral hygiene in patients following stroke. Cochrane Database Syst Rev 2006; 18(4):1–2.

Hypertensive Management

Nicole Thomas, DNP, RN, CCM[1]

KEYWORDS

- Hypertension • Hypertension management • Cerebrovascular accident
- Blood pressure • Hypertensive

KEY POINTS

- Ineffective hypertension management is a key factor in the development of cardiovascular disease.
- The management of hypertension is influenced by personal, behavioral, and health factors.
- Effective management of hypertension is not a linear approach, and patient-specific interventions should be implemented to mitigate the development of chronic diseases caused by ineffective hypertension management.

INTRODUCTION

Hypertension, also known as a key element in the development of cerebrovascular accident (CVA) or stroke, affects 1 in 3 Americans (**Figs. 1** and **2**). Defined as a systolic blood pressure greater than 140 mm Hg and/or a diastolic blood pressure of 90 mm Hg or greater by the American Heart Association (AHA), hypertension is the leading cause of inpatient hospital admits in the United States (US). Accounting for approximately 900,000 inpatient admits and 5000 deaths within the US from 2002 to 2014, hypertensive crisis is a global health problem. Moreover, high blood pressure is responsible for approximately 54% of all strokes, 47% of all ischemic heart disease, and disabling more than 100 million Americans annually.[1,2]

Although this widely used definition of hypertension is essential in overall effective management, it is important to understand other key indications that also define hypertension to ensure a robust approach when managing hypertension. For example, normal high-blood pressure is characterized when an individual who chronically has higher blood pressure readings as a baseline, yet they can still benefit from hypertension management interventions because elevated blood pressures as a normal reading still poses a strain on other essential organs. With normal high-blood pressure, it is critical to keep in mind that the implementation of intervention should be slow and

Louisiana State University Health Science Center School of Nursing, 11120 North Bayou View Drive, Gonzales, LA 70737, USA
[1] Present address: 1900 Gravier St, New Orleans, LA 70002.
E-mail address: Nisaac@lsuhsc.edu

Crit Care Nurs Clin N Am 35 (2023) 31–38
https://doi.org/10.1016/j.cnc.2022.11.001
0899-5885/23/© 2022 Elsevier Inc. All rights reserved.

BLOOD PRESSURE CATEGORY	SYSTOLIC mm Hg (upper number)		DIASTOLIC mm Hg (lower number)
NORMAL	LESS THAN 120	and	LESS THAN 80
ELEVATED	120–129	and	LESS THAN 80
HIGH BLOOD PRESSURE (HYPERTENSION) STAGE 1	130–139	or	80–89
HIGH BLOOD PRESSURE (HYPERTENSION) STAGE 2	140 OR HIGHER	or	90 OR HIGHER
HYPERTENSIVE CRISIS (consult your doctor immediately)	HIGHER THAN 180	and/or	HIGHER THAN 120

Fig. 1. Blood pressure categories. (*Reprinted with permission* https://www.heart.org/-/media/Health-Topics-Images/HBP/blood-pressure-readings-chart-English.jpg. © American Heart Association, Inc.)

steady versus rapid and quick because lowering chronically high-blood pressure can have a significant influence on patients. Finally, there is also isolated systolic hypertension, which is classified as having an elevated systolic blood pressure of greater than 140 mm Hg, yet the diastolic blood pressure is within normal range of less than 90 mm Hg. In isolated systolic hypertension, effective management is still important despite the diastolic blood pressure reading being normal because cardiac disease, kidney disease, and strokes can still occur.[3,4]

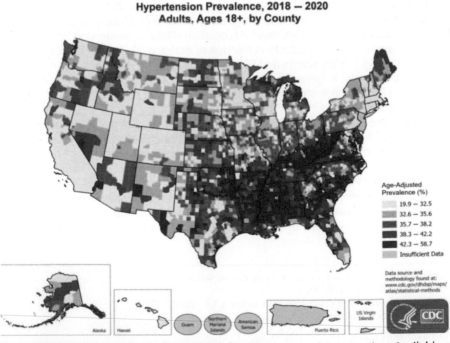

Fig. 2. Hypertension prevalence. (*From* Center for Disease Control & Prevention. Available at https://www.cdc.gov/bloodpressure/facts.htm.)

Despite a decrease in overall inpatient admits and deaths related to strokes that results from hypertension, the overall management of hypertension continues to present significant challenges for the health-care system. Some of the challenges surrounding the effective management of hypertension include but are not limited to obesity, poor lifestyle management such as diet and exercise, increased stress levels, a lack of self-efficacy, and medication adherence. According to an earlier study,[5] the management of hypertension has influencing factors that can be segmented into personal characteristics such as age and gender; socioeconomic background; and behavioral characteristics such as smoking, drinking, lack of exercise, diet, and finally health characteristics such as body mass index, cholesterol levels, insulin levels. The combination of these elements interconnects and relates to each other and thus has a significant influence of the overall management of hypertension.

DISCUSSION

The management of hypertension continues to pose barriers within the health-care system. Effective management of hypertension to mitigate the chronic diseases that result from ineffective hypertension management such as coronary artery disease, kidney disease, and more prominently cerebrovascular disease is obtainable through evidence-based guidelines. With a common mission to address national and global challenges surrounding hypertension management, various health organizations provide clinical guidance, which is based on factual evidence to manage hypertension from personal, socioeconomic, and health perspectives.

The International Society of Hypertension (ISH) provides guidelines that aim to decrease the global burden of hypertension and improve hypertension management from a clinical point of view.[3] In 2020, the ISH's objective was to develop evidence-based guidelines used by clinicians to identify best practices that served as minimum management standards in the effective management of hypertension. These guidelines included the following:

a. Blood pressure reading with systolic greater than 140 mm Hg and diastolic greater than 90 mm Hg × 2 require initial antihypertensive pharmacologic intervention.
b. Patients on antihypertensive medications must have a lipid panel, Hemoglobin (Hgb) A1C, kidney function, and insulin levels drawn quarterly for the first 12 months after being placed on antihypertensive medications and then annually.
c. Blood pressure monitoring is recommended by the patient at least 4 times weekly with parameters provided to the patient as to when to contact their provider for potential further intervention.
d. Lifestyle modifications such as decreasing sodium intake, consuming a low-fat diet, and starting on an exercise regimen.

ISH developed minimum hypertension management standards, and these standards are merely a starting place to mitigate hypertension-mediated organ damage, also known as HMOD, which can be an end-result of untreated hypertension. HMOD is a deviation of the arterial vasculature and/or the organs it supplies that is caused by hypertension.[3] According to an earlier study,[3] despite the implementation of these guidelines, it is important to understand that patients who are already experiencing HMOD may be unlikely to benefit from the minimal standard guidelines from the perspective of developing chronic conditions such as CVA or stroke but these guidelines can, in fact, provide effective guidance on the overall management of patients with hypertension who also have low-to-moderate overall risk through reclassification due to presence of HMOD and influence pharmacologic interventions.

Hypertension-Mediated Organ Damage

The correlation between hypertension and HMOD is relational in the effective management of hypertension. Although hypertension is a disease process that can cause various effects on the human body, the management of hypertension can mitigate those effects and improve overall patient health-care outcomes. Let us discuss some important screenings that should be a part of the plan or care to reduce the risk of developing HMOD. CVAs and transischemic attacks (TIAs) are common results of uncontrolled hypertension. First, any changes to elements of the brain that can indicate a CVA or TIA is occurring such as white matter lesions, infarcts, or atrophy in the brain that are being impacted because of elevated blood pressure can be assessed using an MRI and should be used as a screening tool for patients that present clinically with altered mental status (AMS), changes in cognition, and/or forgetfulness. Second, getting a baseline and then comparative analysis of the electrical activity of the heart is vital. Used as a routine screening tool for patients with a diagnosis of hypertension whom we want to prevent HMOD such as CVA, a 12-lead electrocardiogram allows for an assessment of the electrical activity that can cause critical arrhythmias, which can lead to a heart attack. Third, due to the significant relationship the heart and kidneys have from a pathophysiology perspective, kidney disease, both acute and chronic, should be assessed. Collecting blood specimens to assess the renal function with focus on the serum creatinine and Estimate Glomerular Filtration Rate (eGFR) should be reviewed to determine any potential damage to the function of the renal system. Finally, the arteries are often the most vulnerable organs to the ineffective management of hypertension due to the arterial system that is responsible for the flow of blood, which includes the regulation of the volume and pressure, both high and low. Due to this, obtaining lipid panels that can provide insight as to the plaque buildup within arteries that may be causing elevated blood pressure is important.

Hypertensive Emergencies

Responsible for nearly 35% of all hospital admits, hypertensive emergencies result from a systolic blood pressure greater than 180 mm Hg and/or a diastolic blood pressure of greater than 120 mm Hg with presenting clinical evidence of organ failure. Although multiple organs are at risk for severe injury related to a hypertensive emergency, the heart, kidneys, brain, and arteries are of prominent concern due to the risk of major organ failure that can lead to death. Hypertensive emergencies are considered a medical emergency and must be treated promptly depending on the magnitude of damage caused by crisis.[3] Clinical findings observed in hypertensive crisis include the following:

- Malignant hypertension: Classified as a systolic blood pressure of greater than 200 mm Hg and a diastolic blood pressure of greater than 120 mm Hg, patients often present with blurry vision, AMS, irritability, fatigue, nausea and vomiting, and complaints of chest pain. Treatment plans consist of, but is not limited to, kidney function test, ECG, and a chest radiograph to determine organ damage for appropriate medication treatment. In addition, intravenous blood pressure medications are administered to reduce both systolic and diastolic blood pressure.
- Hypertensive encephalopathy: classified as severely elevated systolic and/or diastolic blood pressure, patients often present with headache, visual disturbances, convulsions, and AMS. Treatment consists of, but is not limited to, addressing the underlying cause, rapidly decreasing the blood pressure, anticonvulsants medications, and vasodilators.

- Hypertensive thrombotic microangiopathy (TMA): also known as TMA is classified as an elevated systolic and/or diastolic blood pressure with hemolysis and thrombocytopenia. Treatment consists of, but is not limited to, lowering the blood pressure with pharmacologic intervention and treating thrombocytopenia.
- An earlier study[3] indicates other clinical presentations of hypertensive crisis, such as cerebral hemorrhage, acute stroke, acute coronary syndrome, cardiogenic pulmonary edema, and aortic aneurysm/dissection, which should be thoroughly assessed and treated accordingly.

Hypertensive emergencies are not the same for all patients who present with severely elevated blood pressure, requiring careful and focused assessments to properly identify issues for rapid and effective intervention.

Hypertension Management and Medication Therapy

The objective of effective hypertension management is to have a systolic blood pressure of less than 140 mm Hg and a diastolic blood pressure of less than 90 mm Hg, with these reading being lower by up to 10 mm Hg for both systolic and diastolic blood pressure in patients that currently have or who are at a higher risk for HMOD. Although management of hypertension can be achieved from a multifaceted approach, pharmacologic interventions are an essential factor in effective management. Various medications are used to effectively manage hypertension with some medications being implemented before others in an effort to start with the most effective low dose, minimal side-effect medications first. Some of the initial first-line medications used in the management of hypertension include beta-blockers, calcium channel blockers, diuretics, angiotensin-converting enzymes, also known as ACE inhibitors, or angiotensin receptor blockers (ARBs). Depending on the overall health status of the patient, such as kidney function, lipid studies, and insulin levels, some patients require 2[6–11] or more antihypertensive medications to effectively manage their blood pressure. Another vital consideration in using pharmacologic therapy to manage hypertension is the need to or if they have blood pressure readings that are greater than 20 mm Hg for systolic blood pressure and greater than 10 mm Hg for diastolic blood pressure.

Diuretics are one of the first-line medications often used in the treatment of hypertension and fall into 3 categories, which includes thiazides, loop, and potassium-sparing diuretics. The mechanism of action for thiazides works through promoting diuresis by inhibiting sodium and chloride cotransporter, which is in the distal convoluted tubule of a nephron. The decrease in sodium reabsorption causes an increase in fluid loss in urine, which subsequently decreases extracellular fluid and plasma volume. The end result is a decrease in overall cardiac output and lowered blood pressure. It is important to remember that because thiazides cause a decrease in potassium and an increase in calcium, frequent laboratory work and supplements may be needed for potassium loss while retaining calcium.

In contrast to thiazides, loop diuretics act on the thick ascending loop of Henle, which is a different anatomic location of the kidney. However, similarly to thiazides, loop diuretics cause diuresis from the urinary system, which causes a decrease in cardiac output resulting in a lowered blood pressure. For patients who are taking loop, please be aware of the potassium loss that corresponds with this medication and the need to potassium laboratories on a frequent basis and potassium supplements.

The final class of diuretics includes potassium-sparing diuretics. The mechanism of action for potassium-sparing diuretics includes the decrease of sodium reabsorption through blocking aldosterone receptors or by inhibiting sodium influx through epithelium sodium-ion channels. It is through the increase of fluid via diuresis that patients experience a decrease in volume, which causes a decline on the demand of the heart, lowering blood pressure.

Another class of medications used in the management of hypertension is antihypertensives, which comes in various forms. One form of antihypertensive medications includes angiotensin-converting enzyme or ACE inhibitors. ACE inhibitors work by relaxing the veins and arteries to lower blood pressure. This is done by stopping the inactive angiotensin I from converting to angiotensin II. By inhibiting the conversion to angiotensin II, narrowing of blood vessels throughout is not achieved and the body lowers the blood pressure. Some examples of ACE inhibitors include

- Benazepril (Lotensin)
- Captopril
- Enalapril (Vasotec)
- Fosinopril
- Lisinopril (Prinivil, Zestril)
- Moexipril
- Perindopril
- Quinapril (Accupril)
- Ramipril (Altace)
- Trandolapril

Alternatively, ARB medication works by blocking angiotensin II from binding to its receptor, which similarly to ACE inhibitors, prevent the narrowing of blood vessels. Although the overall mechanism of action is similar in ACE inhibitors and ARBs, it is important to remember that they work on different elements of the body. Some examples of ARBs include

- Candesartan (Atacand)
- Eprosartan (Teveten),
- Irbesartan (Avapro)
- Losartan (Cozaar)
- Olmesartan (Benicar)
- Telmisartan (Micardis)
- Valsartan (Diovan)

Next, are calcium channel blockers. This antihypertensive medication prevents calcium from entering the muscles, which causes a reduction in contractility within the body, this decreasing the workload of the heart and lowering blood pressure. One of the key functions of calcium within the body is muscle contraction. When muscles contract, flow of blood cannot occur, which is why the inhibiting calcium can aid in effective hypertension management. Some examples of calcium channel blockers include

- Amlodipine (Norvasc)
- Felodipine (Plendil)
- Isradipine (DynaCirc)
- Nicardipine (Cardene)
- Nifedipine (Adalat, Procardia)
- Nimodipine (Nimotop, Nymalize)
- Nisoldipine (Sular)

There are several other types of antihypertensives, the final one we will discuss are beta-blockers. This medication blocks beta-1 adrenergic receptors resulting in slower heart rate, decreased cardiac contractility, and reduced cardiac output. Similar to ACE inhibitors and ARBs, beta blockers can also inhibit the release of angiotensin II, which is responsible for narrowing of blood vessels. The ultimate end result of beta-blockers is lowered blood pressure. Examples of beta-blockers include

- Acebutolol (Sectral)
- Atenolol (Tenormin)
- Betaxolol (Kerlone)
- Bisoprolol (Zebeta, Ziac)
- Carteolol (Cartrol)
- Carvedilol (Coreg)
- Labetalol (Normodyne, Trandate)
- Metoprolol (Lopressor, Toprol-XL)

Therapeutic medication management is an optimal method to control hypertension. In fact, the implementation of a pharmacologic intervention to address hypertension has been the most widely used plan to treat hypertension in all Americans, ultimately lowering diastolic blood pressure by roughly 6 mm Hg in the average American.[12–14] However, adherence to the prescribed medication regimen is another element that should be considered in managing the condition. Medication adherence or lack of adherence can derail the implemented treatment plan if medications are not taken as prescribed. The use of self-efficacy is a strategy that can be used in increasing medication adherence. Self-efficacy, a social cognitive theory, categorized as a human being's level of assurance that they can master the ability to control their actions through education, empowerment, and advocacy has been credited for its success in the effective management of hypertension[6]; Moradi and colleagues, in 2019,[15] conducted a study among 612 patients to determine the effectiveness of self-efficacy in managing hypertension by using the mean self-efficacy score of 2.18. The results of this study made a clear correlation between those individuals whose blood pressure was controlled versus those whose blood pressure was uncontrolled and their self-efficacy score. For example, the average self-efficacy score for those patients with controlled hypertension was 2.30, whereas those with uncontrolled hypertension had a score of 1.83.[12]

Hypertension Management and Lifestyle Modifications

The management of hypertension is not a one-size-fit-all or a linear approach. The multiprong approach that is taken to effectively manage hypertension and mitigate HMOD includes lifestyle modifications such as diet, exercise, smoking cessation, and stress management. The inclusion of lifestyle modifications in the overall treatment plan for managing hypertension is important for longevity and sustainability. Although medication therapy is highly effective, adding 30-minutes or cardio 2 to 3 times per week can result in significant improvements in overall health and the management of hypertension serves as a byproduct of the modification. Another proven lifestyle modification that not only helps to improve hypertension but also helps with overall health is the incorporation of the Dietary Approaches to Stop Hypertension better known as DASH diet. The DASH diet is rich in plant-based foods such as vegetables, grains, and fruits and limited to daily sodium intake to approximately 2 g per day.

SUMMARY

Hypertension affects 1 in 3 Americans and is responsible for more than 900,000 inpatient admits annually. Nearly 47% of all CVAs or strokes occur because of ineffective management of hypertension. Nonetheless, there are clinical interventions that exist to aid in the effective management of hypertension and decrease HMOD such stroke. The most effective and common interventions to mitigate severe complications related to uncontrolled hypertension include pharmacologic regimens, lifestyle modifications, and self-efficacy. The implementation of these interventions can improve hypertension management by almost 37%.

DISCLOSURE

Financial—The author has no fiscal interests in the authorship of the content provided. No compensation or royalty will be provided. Nonfinancial—The author has no conflict of interest in the authorship of the content provided.

REFERENCES

1. Olsen M, Spencer S. A Global perspective of hypertension. Lancet Comm 2015; 386(9994):637–8.
2. Timmermans S, Abdul-Hamid M, Vanderlocht J, et al. Patients with hypertension-associated thrombotic microangiopathy may present with complement abnormalities. Kidney Int 2017;91(6):1420–5.
3. Unger T, Borghi C, Charchar F, et al. International Society of Hypertension global hypertension practice guidelines. J Hypertens 2020;38(6):982–1004.
4. Warren-Findlow J, Seymour RB, Brunner Huber LR. The association between self-efficacy and hypertension self-care activities among African American adults. J Community Health 2012;37(1):15–24.
5. Wu Y, Ma G, Feng N, et al. The pathogenesis and influencing factors of adult hypertension based on structural equation Scanning. Scanning 2022;2022: 2663604.
6. American Psychological Association. Teaching tip sheet self-efficacy. 2019. Retrieved from. https://www.apa.org/pi/aids/resources/education/self-efficacy.
7. Center for Disease Control and Prevention. High blood pressure. 2019. Retrieved from. https://www.cdc.gov/bloodpressure/index.htm.
8. Chakraborty D, Choudhury S, Lahiry S. Hypertension clinical practice guidelines (ISH, 2020): what is new? Med Princ Pract 2021;30(6):579–84.
9. Hallberg I, Ranerup A, Kjellgren K. Supporting the self-management of hypertension: patient's experiences of using a mobile phone-based system. J Hum Hypertens 2016;30(2):141–6.
10. Journal of Cardiovascular Nursing. About the journal. 2020. Retrieved from. https://journals.lww.com/jcnjournal/Pages/aboutthejournal.aspx.
11. Lackland D. Racial differences in hypertension: implications for high blood pressure management. Am J Med Sci 2014;348(2):135–8.
12. Najimi A, Mostafavi F, Sharifirad G, et al. Development and study of self-efficacy scale in medication adherence among Iranian patients with hypertension. J Education Health Promotion 2017;6:83.
13. Nguyen Q, Dominguez J, Nguyen L, et al. Hypertension management: an update. Am Health Drug Benefits 2010;3(1):47–56.
14. Petiprin A. Health behavioral theory. 2016. Retrieved from. http://nursing-theory.org/theories- and-models/Johnson-behavior-system-model.php.
15. Moradi M, Nasiri M, Jahanshahi M, et al. The effects of a self- management program based on the 5 A's model on self-efficacy among older men with hypertension. Nurse Midwifery Studies 2019;8(1):21–7.

Nursing Management of Temperature in a Patient with Stroke

Kristine M. McGlennen, DNP, APRN[a,1,]*,
Gemi E. Jannotta, PhD, APRN[a,1], Sarah L. Livesay, DNP, APRN, FNCS[b,1]

KEYWORDS

- Targeted temperature management (TTM) • Therapeutic hypothermia (TH) • Stroke
- Fever • Controlled normothermia • Nursing intervention • Fever monitoring

KEY POINTS

- Fever is common in stroke and is associated with poor neurological outcomes.
- Targeted temperature management (TTM) may improve the monitoring and management of fever, thereby mitigating risk of secondary brain injury; however, the clinical utility of this intervention in patients with stroke is unknown due to insufficient research.
- Nurses are invaluable and aid in the prompt identification, treatment, and management of fever. They should be knowledgeable about the current evidence around TTM and stroke, temperature monitoring devices, complications, and various nursing interventions to deliver exceptional stroke care.

INTRODUCTION

Over the past several decades, medical and nursing studies explored the relationship between brain injury and temperature. Studies in the early 2000s suggested that inducing mild hypothermia in patients with hypoxic ischemic injury after cardiac arrest was associated with improved neurologic outcome, and these findings inspired additional trials in multiple areas of brain injury including stroke.[1] Over the past 5 years, several research studies continued to shape the management of temperature in patients with hypoxic-ischemic injury, and the nursing and medical management of these patients shifted from induced hypothermia to a focus on fever prevention and targeted temperature management (TTM).[2] Temperature management (TM) remains a key nursing issue in the acute care of patients with all types of stroke, including acute ischemic stroke (AIS), intracranial hemorrhage (ICH), and

[a] Department of Anesthesia and Pain Medicine, University of Washington; [b] Department of Anesthesia and Pain Medicine, University of Washington, Rush University College of Nursing
[1] Present address: Harborbview Medical Center, Neurocritical Care, 325 9th Avenue, Seattle, WA 98104.
* Corresponding author. Harborbview Medical Center, Neurocritical Care, 325 9th Avenue, Seattle, WA 98104.
E-mail address: kmcglenn@uw.edu

Crit Care Nurs Clin N Am 35 (2023) 39–52
https://doi.org/10.1016/j.cnc.2022.10.005
0899-5885/23/© 2022 Elsevier Inc. All rights reserved.

Abbreviations	
TTM	Targeted Temperature Managament
TC	Temperature Control
TM	Temperature Managment
EBP	Evidence Based Practice
AIS	Acute Ischemic Stroke
ICH	Intracranial Hemorrhage
aSAH	Aneurysmal Subarachnoid Hemorrhage
ICU	Intensive Care Unit
TBI	Traumatic Brain Injury
LOS	Length of stay
IVH	Intraventricular hemorrhage
DCI	Delayed cerebral ischemia
RTC	Randomized controlled trials
TH	Theraputic Hypothermia
PHE	Perihematomal edema
ICP	Intracranial pressure
RTD	Resistive temperature detectors
EKG	Electrocardiogram

aneurysmal subarachnoid hemorrhage (aSAH). However, the indications for intervention, duration of management, and targeted temperature differ in the stroke population. This article reviews the literature and synthesizes the nursing management of temperature in patients with stroke, focusing on the highest acuity patients receiving care in the intensive care unit (ICU).

TARGETED TEMPERATURE MANAGEMENT DEFINED

The nomenclature for temperature control (TC) in brain injury has changed over the years as the studies supporting the manipulation of temperature have evolved. Induced hypothermia is generally categorized as mild when the body temperature is controlled to 33°C to 36°C and moderate or extreme if the body temperature dropped below 32°C. However, the term induced hypothermia did not address interventions to control fever and control body temperature to normothermia. Therefore, the term TTM was largely adopted to reflect both induced hypothermia and measures to control fever in patients with brain injury. Current articles generally use either the term TTM or TC to indicate the wide variety of interventions to control body temperature across a range of goal temperatures in patients with brain injury.

TEMPERATURE IN BRAIN INJURY

Following a neurological injury, the brain is susceptible to secondary damage from ischemia, edema, and alterations in cerebral metabolism.[3] Fever, which is very common among individuals with neurologic injuries, increases susceptibility to subsequent neurological injury. The underlying cause of thermal dysregulation after neurological insult is not well understood, in part, due to the heterogeneity of the underlying pathophysiology of brain injury subtypes (eg, traumatic brain injury [TBI], AIS, ICH, and aSAH).[1,4] Various interrelated mechanisms have been cited as precipitating neurogenic fever including damage to the hypothalamus, alterations in cerebral blood flow (eg, vasospasm) and metabolism, impaired heat dispersion, a surge of proinflammatory substances (eg, cytokines), and blood product degradation. Infectious etiology is also common and accounts for a large proportion of fevers in neurocritical care.[1] Although it can be challenging to discern between infectious and neurogenic fevers,[5] regardless of its etiology, fever should be avoided in brain injury.

FEVER IN ISCHEMIC AND HEMORRHAGIC STROKE

Pyrexia is common after all types of stroke and is associated with worse clinical outcomes,[4,6–9] including longer length of stay (LOS),[4,7,9] higher mortality,[7,9,10] and disability.[4,7,9,10] The association between fever and poor functional outcomes is not well understood.[1,11] Hyperthermia is thought to precipitate secondary injury by increasing metabolic demand (thereby increasing cerebral oxygen consumption), inducing a pro-inflammatory cytokine surge and exacerbating blood-brain barrier disruption[8]; however, we cannot exclude the possibility that fever, instead of inciting neurological sequelae, may itself be a symptom of a related but independent critical event.[11]

Acute Ischemic Stroke

Pyrexia is a frequent complication of AIS, affecting approximately 50% of patients.[12] Early fever (ie, fever within the first 24 hours) is particularly common in this patient population and is associated with worse outcomes.[1] In fact, the Copenhagen Stroke study demonstrated a 30% higher risk of mortality for patients with increased body temperature (eg, >1°C) on admission.[4] This association between early fever and mortality was later corroborated by a meta-analysis, which demonstrated a nearly 2-fold higher rate of mortality among AIS patients with early fever regardless of age or stroke severity.[4] Collectively, this underscores the importance of fever prevention in patients with AIS, as fever portends worse clinical outcomes.

Intracranial Hemorrhage

The overall prevalence and underlying pathophysiology of hyperthermia in ICH remains uncertain due to a lack of clinical trials. Fever among patients with spontaneous ICH is associated with hematoma expansion,[6,13] cerebral edema,[6] and poor neurological outcomes.[6] Delayed fever (>24 hours after admission) is more common among patients with ICH; however, pyrexia within 24 hours of admission and sustained fever (ie, >72 hours) is associated with disproportionately worse outcomes.[4] Individuals with a large ICH volume, intraventricular hemorrhage (IVH), and/or deep location of bleed have a higher propensity toward fever development.[13] Gillow and colleagues[13] also noted pyrexia to be more common among patients who received neurosurgical interventions such as extraventricular drain insertion or craniotomy with hematoma evacuation. Expert consensus recommends TTM (36.5°C–37.5°C) for patient with ICH who have noninfectious fevers[10]; however, it is unclear whether this intervention offers any clinical benefit[6,14] and may be associated with unintended consequences such as increased LOS and time on mechanical ventilator.[14]

Aneurysmal Subarachnoid Hemorrhage

Hyperthermia is extremely common in aSAH, affecting as many as 70% of patients within the first 10 days of injury,[15] and is associated with delayed cerebral ischemia (DCI),[5] increased mortality,[1,4,5] and disability.[4,5] The association between fever and neurological outcomes is more complex in this population due to interrelated complications including IVH, DCI, and vasospasm.[4] Severe aSAH and IVH are risk factors for refractory fever.[4,11,15] Furthermore, patients with symptomatic vasospasm are more likely to develop hyperthermia, which is suggestive of a common underlying etiology for both phenomena.[4,11] Irrespective of the underlying pathophysiology, pyrexia after aSAH is associated with heightened ischemia, increased edema, and elevated intracranial pressure (ICP), which collectively can precipitate secondary brain injury and decreased level of consciousness.[11] Prompt identification and treatment of fever is therefore critical to preventing neurological sequelae.[4,11] Pyrexia mitigation through targeted temperature regulation (ie, normothermia) is recommended to prevent secondary brain injury; however, this recommendation comes largely from expert opinion, as Randomized control trials (RCTs) are lacking. Although fever control measures (eg, cooling devices and antipyretics) have been shown to reduce fever burden in aSAH, there is no significant difference in functional outcomes, making this recommendation more theoretical than data-driven.[16]

Despite considerable variability in timing, effects, and underlying pathophysiology of fever among the multiple stroke subtypes, it is well established that fever is harmful and exacerbates neuronal injury in all stroke types.[4] Active TM or reduction of body temperature to normothermia may be a neuroprotective strategy for stroke patients[3,6,15–18]; however, the utility of this intervention is largely suppositious as high grade evidence is lacking.[16] In the absence of robust data to support the role of TTM in stroke, expert consensus holds that fever control should be the standard of care[7,16,18–20] due to its potential to mitigate secondary injury.

HYPOTHERMIA IN ISCHEMIC AND HEMORRHAGIC STROKE

Existing literature shows a benefit of therapeutic hypothermia (TH) in instances of global hypoperfusion (ie, post-cardiac arrest) but remains inconclusive whether hypothermia confers neurological benefit for other distinct neurological processes such as ICH, aSAH, and AIS. Owing to the distinct pathophysiological pathways and multimodal effects of TTM, it is difficult to generalize the effects of temperature modulation on specific intracranial pathologies.[6] It is posited that hypothermia may provide neuroprotection by reducing energy consumption, free radical protection, and inflammation.[15]

Acute Ischemic Stroke

There is a paucity of large, multicenter clinical trials investigating the impact of hypothermia on mortality and clinical outcomes in AIS[4]; thus, it is unknown whether TH confers any benefit in AIS.[4,8,12,20] Most of the existing clinical trials are quasi-experimental or small pilot trials, which aimed to determine the feasibility and safety profile of TH. In particular, a series of pilot studies conducted by Schwab and colleagues investigated TH on elevated ICP in patients with large middle cerebral artery (MCA) stroke and cerebral edema (also known as malignant MCA syndrome). Investigators demonstrated decreased ICP during the initial stage of TH (33°C), however, this effect was transient and the rewarming phase led to excessive rebound elevations in ICP which was associated with increased mortality.[4] The few existing RCTs have found no benefit of TH on ischemic stroke outcomes[4,8,12,21]; however, these studies are underpowered and limited by small sample sizes.[4,8] Several meta-analyses have emerged in an effort to increase power and better evaluate the impact of hypothermia on AIS outcomes; collectively, these analyses found no significant difference in function outcomes. Furthermore, one analysis suggested higher mortality among patients treated with TH.[4] Finally, a retrospective study by Choi and colleagues demonstrated differential effects of TTM among patients with AIS who received treatment with endovascular thrombectomy. Patients with AIS who underwent TTM (cooled to 34.5°C) were more likely to have disability than those who received standard of care. However, individuals with a higher risk of a poor outcome (ie, large ischemic core, minimal viable penumbra, and/or NIHSS >20) were less likely to have hemorrhagic conversion and therefore had a more favorable outcome if they were treated with TTM compared with standard of care. TTM was associated with a higher prevalence of major complications (eg, pneumonia, bradycardia, pressure injuries) than those treated with standard of care,[21] underscoring the importance of additional research to inform risk benefit decisions. Larger RCTs are warranted to better evaluate the safety profile and role of TH patients with AIS. At this time, TH is not generally offered in this patient population.

Intracranial Hemorrhage

TH has been shown to reduce edema, decrease inflammation, and minimize the disruption of blood-brain barrier in animal models of ICH; however, it remains unclear whether TH in humans with spontaneous ICH offers any morbidity and mortality benefit due to a lack of clinical trials[4,6] and contradictory findings among the few existing clinical trials. Specifically, one small pilot study found that mild TH (reduced core temperature to 35°C for 10 days) led to a reduction of perihematoma edema (PHE) and led to improved functional outcomes.[6] However, another small, retrospective case study conducted by Volbers and colleagues[22] demonstrated that although early TH led to an initial reduction in PHE, after 3 days, there was no difference in PHE or clinical outcomes. In light of the limited, contradictory evidence, TH is avoided in this patient population.

Aneurysmal Subarachnoid Hemorrhage

Fever is common in aSAH and is associated with delayed DCI and worse neurological outcomes.[5] Although TH has been shown to be neuroprotective in animal models, existing human literature fails to demonstrate any definitive benefit on neurological outcomes, refractory intracranial hypertension, and/or vasospasm incidence.[4] Existing literature is limited to small, non-randomized clinical trials that are inadequately powered[4,23] but offer preliminary evidence in favor of TH for aSAH. A series of small studies have demonstrated that TH improves neurological recovery in patients undergoing aneurysmal clipping and confers neuroprotection in poor grade aSAH patients by decreasing incidence of vasospasm and DCI.[24] Furthermore, a recent retrospective study conducted by Won and colleagues[23] demonstrated a significant decrease in mortality and cerebral edema in aSAH patients treated with hypothermia compared with the standard of care with no difference in complication rates.

TH is not generally offered proactively to improve outcomes in this patients with aSAH; however, TH is used for patients with ICP crisis that is refractory to other medical management. Although the data for this intervention are most robust in patients with TBI, this intervention is applied to patients with hemorrhagic strokes as a part of ICP management pathways. When used in this context, TH is generally effective at reducing ICP but is not associated with improved neurologic outcome in patients with TBI.[25] Elevated ICP that is refractory to medical management in a patient with ICH or aSAH may be an occasion when TH is used as a tool to manage ICP in patients with stroke.

NURSING MANAGEMENT OF TEMPERATURE IN STROKE

Armed with the knowledge of the frequency and impact of fever in stroke patients, the bedside nurse is key to monitoring temperature and working with the health care team to intervene accordingly.

Monitoring of Fever in Patients with Stroke

The deleterious effects of hyperthermia in stroke patients are well documented; yet, fever remains undertreated due to a lack of consensus regarding the temperature threshold at which to initiate TTM and standardized guidelines for patient monitoring and TM.[7,19,20] For example, the American Heart Association and American Stroke Association's stroke guidelines recommend prompt treatment of fever (>38°C) with antipyretics but does not specify pharmacologic agents nor advocate for more aggressive temperature regulation with TTM.[4,20] The lack of formalized guidelines stems from a dearth of clinical trials, as current recommendations are informed largely by case studies[12] and expert consensus.[10,12] However, given the data suggesting worse outcomes in patients with all types of stroke and fever, nursing should monitor temperature diligently, notify the provider when temperature exceeds 38°C and intervene promptly. General consensus recommends TTM initiation when temperature exceed 37.5°C with a targeted range of 36.5°C to 37.5°C.[18]

Nurses play a crucial role in the identification and treatment of fever.[7,17,19] Temperature monitoring is a routine observation obtained by the bedside nurse, which provides valuable information about a patients' condition, leading to important decisions regarding investigations and treatments.[26] There are many technologies currently being uses to monitor temperature including resistive temperature detectors (RTDs), thermally sensitive resistors (thermistors), mercury thermometers, noncontact infrared thermometers, thermocouple sensors, field-effect transistors, optical sensors as well as luminescent materials.[27]

Nursing standards of practice for temperature monitoring vary by institution as do the devices that are used to obtain temperature measurements. There are many sites used to monitor temperature in the ICU and each site has clinical considerations that should be evaluated and managed by the bedside nurse. **Table 1** is a summary of the most common sites and technology used to obtain temperature along with clinical considerations for the bedside nurse. Historically, the highest standard for temperature monitoring accuracy has been via the pulmonary artery catheter. However, utilization of these catheters is dwindling therefore esophageal and bladder probes have been deemed the "next best" measurements.[3] When fever is detected, nursing should promptly institute TTM interventions and ensure continuous core temperature monitoring.[4,17,18,20,28] If core temperature monitoring is not possible, temperature should be obtained via oral or tympanic route[19] at least every hour.[18] Temporal and axillary routes are the least preferred route for temperature monitoring for patients with stroke in the most acute phase of their illness as they are often inaccurate and may result in the under-recognition of pyrexia.[3,19]

TTM is a broad term for a number of nursing and medical interventions aimed at decreasing fever or inducing hypothermia depending on the clinical situation. The interventions range in intensity from administering an antipyretic such as acetaminophen, applying fans or ice packs, and cooling the room temperature to applying advanced cooling technology (surface cooling, gel cooling pads, and intravenous cooling catheters).[3]

When less aggressive interventions such as antipyretic medications or cooled room are not effective at controlling fever, the nurse may be asked to use advanced cooling devices. When used, the technology is applied with a targeted temperature of 36.5 C to 37.5 C.[18] Although no specific cooling measure has proven superiority, surface cooling measures are often associated with higher temperature deviation.[3,17] High-quality TTM is contingent on vigilant monitoring of the patient's response to treatment and prevention of complications. One of the most common unintended effects of TTM

Table 1
Common temperature sites, types of monitoring devices, and clinical considerations

Site	Type	Clinical Considerations
Axilla	RTD, digital or alcohol thermometer	• Accuracy is affected by sweating, ambient temperature, and incorrect placement of the probe • Typically requires 5–10 min to obtain accurate temperature • Temperature cannot be measured continuously
Bladder	Electrical (thermistors, thermocouples, or RTDs)	• Requires aseptic insertion technique • The cost is more than a regular Foley catheter • Associated with infection
Brain	Electrical (thermistors, thermocouples, or RTDs)	• Accuracy is affected if placed in an area of damaged brain • Must be placed by a neurosurgeon • Extremely invasive
Esophageal	Electrical (thermistors, thermocouples, or RTDs)	• Accuracy is affected by fluids passing through the nasogastric tube and placement • Probe placement should be in the distal third of the esophagus • Position should be confirmed with x-ray
Intravenous	Electrical (thermistors, thermocouples, or RTDs)	• Must be placed by qualified providers only • Pulmonary artery catheters and cooling catheters are infrequently used • Increased risk of infection compared with other sites
Nasopharyngeal	Thermocouples	• Accuracy is affected by probe placement and airflow • Probe placement should be a few centimeters past the nares • There should be obstruction of airflow to avoid cooling the probe
Oral	Alcohol thermometer	• Accuracy is affected by ability to keep mouth closed • Typically requires 5–10 min to obtain accurate temperature • Temperature cannot be measured continuously
Rectal	Electrical (thermistors, thermocouples, or RTDs)	• Accuracy is affected by the presence of feces and position • Probe should be inserted approximately 4 cm into the rectum • Risk of perforation exists
Temporal	Infrared	• Accuracy is affected by ambient air temperature and sweating • Temperature cannot be measured continuously
Tympanic	Infrared	• Accuracy is affected by tortuous ear canal or obstruction by cerumen • Temperature cannot be measured continuously

Abbreviation: RTDs, resistive temperature detectors.

is shivering, which usually occurs when core temperature is less than 36.5 C. Diligent temperature monitoring can help mitigate the risk of iatrogenic shivering and guide interventions to maintain temperature within the targeted range. Finally, the temperature of the cooling device should be monitored closely as it informs clinicians about the patient's response to fever reduction strategies[17] and lower temperatures are associated with higher risk of impaired skin integrity.[29] It is worth noting that although the emphasis of this discussion focuses onTM in the ICU, fever may occur throughout all stages of stroke recovery. The same fever management principles—that is, prompt recognition and treatment—should be applied in any clinical setting (eg., acute care, rehabilitation). Monitoring frequency and interventions may be modified to align with the acuity standards of that particular clinical setting.

Complications of Therapeutic Temperature Management

The most extreme and life-threatening complications associated with TTM occur when the body temperature is dropped below 32°C. At these temperatures, multiple systemic effects may occur including dysrhythmias that are refractory to treatment, significant electrolyte shifts, and dehydration associated with a cold-induced diuresis.[30] Modern TTM does not target a temperature below 33°C. As the goal body temperature increases to the normothermia range, the complications are generally less extreme, although they still require nursing monitoring and management. In patients with stroke, nurses must diligently monitor patients for shivering, skin breakdown, and deep vein thrombosis development depending on cooling technology selected.[3,28,31] See **Table 2**, for common complications associated with TTM and nursing monitoring and suggested interventions.

Shiver Monitoring and Management

Shivering is a normal physiologic response by which the body attempts to produce heat to increase the body temperature. When inducing hypothermia for reasons such as controlling elevated ICP, shivering occurs most commonly and is most rigorous when the body is between 35°C to 36°C.[32] The shivering response decreases as the body temperature drops below 35°C. However, shivering is common any time the body temperature is being reduced from a febrile state and may be common in patients with stroke receiving TTM interventions. Shivering increases the metabolic demand on the body, oxygen metabolism in the brain, and may negate the benefit of controlling the body temperature during brain injury. Therefore, patients receiving TTM should be closely monitored for the presence of shivering and the nursing team should intervene to control shivering as much as possible.[32]

The Bedside Shiver Assessment Scale is a validated tool that all health care providers can use to objectively assess shivering. Patients are first visually observed for shivering, followed by palpation of the muscles on the neck, thorax, arms, and legs. Patients are given a score of 0 to 3 (**Box 1**) to describe the presence of shivering. The score has been successfully used to implement a step-wise, nurse-led protocol to minimize shivering.[33]

The treatment of shivering spans both non-pharmacological and pharmacologic interventions.[32] Surface counter warming of the face, arms, and legs with warm towels or a warming blanket can effectively minimize shivering, whereas the core remains cooled. Oral medications such as acetaminophen and buspirone may alleviate shivering by decreasing the body temperature or lowering the shiver threshold, respectively. Intravenous magnesium to maintain normal to slightly elevated serum magnesium levels may minimize shivering. Sedation in escalating doses and paralytics may be required to effectively control shivering in severe cases. Close

Table 2
Common therapeutic temperature management complications, nursing monitoring, and suggested interventions

Temperature	Complication	Phase of TTM	Nursing Monitoring	Possible Interventions
Mild hypothermia (33°C–36°C)	Cold-induced diuresis	Induction	• Hourly output (particularly during induction)	• IV fluid boluses to maintain euvolemia • Potassium replacement • Other electrolyte replacement as needed
	Intracellular shift of potassium during induction	Induction	• Telemetry monitoring, EKG • Frequent laboratory values (q4hr)	• Caution when replacing potassium prior to or during rewarming • Notify provider immediately if potassium elevated or EKG changes
	Extracellular shift of potassium	Rewarming	• Telemetry monitoring, EKG • Frequent laboratory values (q4hr)	• Slow or stop rewarming • Decrease target temperature
	Rebound cerebral edema, elevated ICP	Rewarming	• Frequent neurologic assessments • Slow and controlled rewarming • Frequent ICP monitoring	
	Decreased GI motility	Throughout	• Tolerance of enteral nutrition • Bowel movement frequency and consistency	• Nutrition consult • Decrease enteral feeding rate • Pro-motility medications
	Insulin resistance	Throughout	• Frequent monitoring of blood glucose levels	• Increased insulin requirements (IV or SQ)
All TTM temperature ranges	Skin breakdown	Throughout; more common with surface cooling	• Frequent skin assessment • Monitoring of water bath temperature	• Treatment of shivering, fever • Repositioning • Stopping TTM if water bath is cold for extended periods of time
	DVT development	Throughout; more common with IV cooling technology	• Monitor for swelling, thrombophlebitis	• DVT prophylaxis
	Shivering	Throughout; more common at 35°C–36°C	• Shiver assessment using a validated tool	• Stepwise approach to shiver control

Abbreviations: DVT, deep venous thrombosis; EKG, electrocardiogram; GI, gastrointestinal; ICP, intracranial pressure; IV, intravenous; q4hr, every 4 hours; SQ, subcutaneous; TTM, therapeutic temperature management.

Box 1
The bedside shiver assessment scale[45]

0—None: no shivering noted on palpation of the masseter, neck, or chest wall

1—Mild: shivering localized to neck and/or thorax only

2—Moderate: shivering involves gross movement of the upper extremities (in addition to neck and thorax)

3—Severe: shivering involves gross movements of the trunk and upper and lower extremities

---

monitoring and treatment of shivering are particularly warranted when TTM is used as an intervention to address elevated ICP that is refractory to other interventions. When TTM is used to address fever in a patient with stroke, the treatment team must weigh the benefits and risk of aggressive fever management that may require escalating doses of sedation, particularly in patients who are not intubated and have a neurologic examination to follow. Current research to assess the risks and benefits of aggressive fever control and shiver management in this population is limited.

Therapeutic Temperature Management and Patient Care Bundles

Fever management is frequently included in care pathways or bundles of nursing interventions for patients with stroke. Care bundles are a set of three to five evidence-based practices (EBPs) performed collectively and reliably to improve the quality of care. Care bundles are used widely across health care settings with the aim of preventing and managing different health conditions.[34] Bundling of EBPs is familiar to nurses and is used to improve patient care and outcomes in a variety of health care settings.[35] Sepsis bundles, central line care bundles, skin care and turning bundles, mouth care and pneumonia prevention bundles, communication for handoff bundles, and the ABCDEF care bundles are examples of only a few bundles in current practice that are nurse-led and have been used to improve the overall care of the hospitalized patient. An elevation of temperature above 37.5 °C is common in patients with stroke[36,37] and is associated with worse outcomes.[38] Avoidance of fever, in combination with glucose control and swallow evaluation, has been identified in international guidelines as priorities for inpatient stroke management.[39,40] Therefore, many stroke programs include fever monitoring and management in standard nursing care bundles for patients with stroke. These bundles should address the application of TTM as well as complications of monitoring and management.[28] Although nursing-led bundles for fever management are common practice, the interventions used and threshold for treatment differ between organizations. More research is needed to understand if the bundle interventions or the presence of a bundle and nursing attention to fever overall improves the recognition and treatment of fever, and if this management improves outcomes for patients with stroke.

LOOKING AHEAD: THE FUTURE OF TEMPERATURE MANAGEMENT IN STROKE

The Impact of Fever Prevention in Brain-Injured Patients (INTREPID) study is a multi-center randomized controlled trail currently underway to understand the impact of aggressive fever management (using surface gel cooling pads known as the Arctic Sun System) in multiple diseases including AIS, ICH, and aSAH. Enrolled patients were randomized to either aggressive fever management to 37°C or standard of care. The study outcomes include total fever burden and neurologic outcome at

3 months measured by modified Rankin Score. The study has completed enrollment, and results are expected in the next year.[9]

Technology advancements continue to change the way nurses interact with their patients and the data obtained from the patient. Recent advances in remote technologies are making their way to the bedside and many believe that the next step in the evolution of vital sign monitoring in the ICU is remote. Several temperature monitors have been released that use a simple device attached to the skin with flexible adherent tape or electrodes similar to electrocardiogram (EKG) leads. Many of these new monitoring techniques are accompanied by technology for remote monitoring with algorithms that are set up to alert nursing staff to acute changes and even suggest treatment options.[41]

The most frequently used techniques to manage temperature in the ICU are primarily managed by the bedside nurse as part of TC bundles. These include antipyretic medications, ice packs, cooling blankets, gel pads, and intra-arterial cooling catheters. Many believe that there is opportunity for new technology to meet the standard of care to keep temperature within normal limits for all patients experiencing stroke. One novel technology for TM is an intranasal cooling system using compressed air to spray perfluorocarbon, a liquid coolant, into the nostrils. This has been developed and tested in Europe (PRINCESS trial), and the company claims that the device is able to lower body temperature several hours sooner than alternative cooling practices.[42] Another device known as ThermoSuit(R) uses thin liquid convection to cool skin directly and is FDA-approved for use in hyperthermia but undergoing phase II trials in stroke patients.[43] The device is similar to a sleeping bag and lies flat on a hospital bed. Cold water is continuously circulated and replenished through the suit at about 14 L/min. The patient stays in the suit for approximately 30 minutes yet its cooling effects can last up to 24 hours after treatment. Finally, there is recent research in the area of selective brain cooling (SBC). SBC is defined as the lowering of the brain temperature either locally or below arterial blood temperature and has been evaluated in animal models and clinical trials. This method has not garnered robust implementation due to some concerns regarding appropriate methods for achieving TM and technical setbacks such as insufficient cooling power, cost and irritating effects on skin, and mucosal interfaces.[44] Further research in this area is required to evaluate the clinical relevance of these new TM techniques.

SUMMARY

Fever is highly prevalent in all types of strokes and is associated with higher LOS, disability, and mortality. TTM or the strategic reduction of body temperature to a specific threshold has emerged as a potential intervention to mitigate neurological sequelae after stroke; however, the research is too limited to draw conclusions about the benefit of TTM for stroke patients. Given the well-recognized deleterious effects of fever after stroke, expert consensus recommends treating fever in all stroke patients. Nurses play an essential role in the early detection, monitoring, and treatment of fever and its complications. Temperature monitoring and normothermia induction may be accomplished through various means. Effective TTM requires bedside nurses to be knowledgeable about the accuracy, clinical considerations, monitoring, and possible interventions associated with each temperature modality and cooling methods. Institution-specific TTM care bundles may also improve TM in patients with stroke. Although the INTREPID trial is underway, TTM in stroke remains under-investigated and warrants large, multicenter RCTs to discern the impact of the intervention on patient outcomes.

CLINICS CARE POINTS

- Pyrexia is common after all types of stroke (AIS, ICH, aSAH) and is associated with worse clinical outcomes, including longer LOS, higher mortality, and disability.
- While the role of TTM in acute management of stroke patients remains understudied, fever prevention is of paramount importance as it is may mitigate secondary injury.
- Nurses play a crucial role in the identification and treatment of fever. While institutional practice variations exist, nurses should promptly institute TTM interventions and ensure continuous core temperature monitoring when a fever is detected.
- High-quality TTM is contingent on vigilant monitoring of the patient's response to treatment and prevention of complications (e.g., shivering, skin breakdown and DVT).
- Use of validated tools, (eg, the Bedside Shiver Assessment Scale) and patient care bundles may aid in the prompt identification of and management of fever and its complications.

REFERENCES

1. Gowda R, Jaffa M, Badjatia N. Thermoregulation in brain injury. Handb Clin Neurol 2018;157:789–97.
2. Morrison LJ, Thoma B. Translating targeted temperature management trials into postarrest care. N Engl J Med 2021;384(24):2344–5.
3. Madden LK, Hill M, May TL, et al. The implementation of targeted temperature management: an evidence-based guideline from the neurocritical care society. Neurocrit Care 2017;27(3):468–87.
4. Marehbian J, Greer DM. Normothermia and stroke. Curr Treat Options Neurol 2017;19(1):4.
5. Rocha Ferreira da Silva I, Rodriguez de Freitas G. Early predictors of fever in patients with aneurysmal subarachnoid hemorrhage. J Stroke Cerebrovasc Dis 2016;25(12):2886–90.
6. Fischer M, Schiefecker A, Lackner P, et al. Targeted temperature management in spontaneous intracerebral hemorrhage: a systematic review. Curr Drug Targets 2017;18(12):1430–40.
7. Thompson HJ, Kagan SH. Clinical management of fever by nurses: doing what works. J Adv Nurs 2011;67(2):359–70.
8. Drewry A, Mohr NM. Temperature management in the ICU. Crit Care Med 2022;50(7):1138–47.
9. Greer DM, Ritter J, Helbok R, et al. Impact of fever prevention in brain-injured patients (INTREPID): study protocol for a randomized controlled trial. Neurocrit Care 2021;35(2):577–89.
10. Andrews PJ, Sinclair HL, Rodríguez A, et al. Therapeutic hypothermia to reduce intracranial pressure after traumatic brain injury: the Eurotherm3235 RCT. Health Technol Assess 2018;22(45):1–134.
11. Scaravilli V, Tinchero G, Citerio G. Fever management in SAH. Neurocrit Care 2011;15(2):287–94.
12. Ntaios G, Dziedzic T, Michel P, et al. European Stroke Organisation (ESO) guidelines for the management of temperature in patients with acute ischemic stroke. Int J Stroke 2015;10(6):941–9.
13. Gillow SJ, Ouyang B, Lee VH, et al. Factors associated with fever in intracerebral hemorrhage. J Stroke Cerebrovasc Dis 2017;26(6):1204–8.
14. Lord AS, Karinja S, Lantigua H, et al. Therapeutic temperature modulation for fever after intracerebral hemorrhage. Neurocrit Care 2014;21(2):200–6.

15. Andresen M, Gazmuri JT, Marín A, et al. Therapeutic hypothermia for acute brain injuries. Scand J Trauma Resusc Emerg Med 2015;23:42.
16. Hall A, O'Kane R. The extracranial consequences of subarachnoid hemorrhage. World Neurosurg 2018;109:381–92.
17. Moreda M, Beacham PS, Reese A, et al. Increasing the effectiveness of targeted temperature management. Crit Care Nurse 2021;41(5):59–63.
18. Andrews PJD, Verma V, Healy M, et al. Targeted temperature management in patients with intracerebral haemorrhage, subarachnoid haemorrhage, or acute ischaemic stroke: consensus recommendations. Br J Anaesth 2018;121(4):768–75.
19. Rockett H, Thompson HJ, Blissitt PA. Fever management practices of neuroscience nurses: what has changed? J Neurosci Nurs 2015;47(2):66–75.
20. Powers WJ, Rabinstein AA, Ackerson T, et al. Guidelines for the early management of patients with acute ischemic stroke: 2019 update to the 2018 guidelines for the early management of acute ischemic stroke: a guideline for healthcare professionals from the American Heart association/American stroke association. Stroke 2019;50(12):e344–418.
21. Choi MH, Gil YE, Lee SJ, et al. The clinical usefulness of targeted temperature management in acute ischemic stroke with malignant trait after endovascular thrombectomy. Neurocrit Care 2021;34(3):990–9.
22. Volbers B, Herrmann S, Willfarth W, et al. Impact of hypothermia initiation and duration on perihemorrhagic edema evolution after intracerebral hemorrhage. Stroke 2016;47(9):2249–55.
23. Won SY, Kim MK, Song J, et al. Therapeutic hypothermia in patients with poor-grade aneurysmal subarachnoid hemorrhage. Clin Neurol Neurosurg 2022;221:107369.
24. Ravishankar N, Nuoman R, Amuluru K, et al. Management strategies for intracranial pressure crises in subarachnoid hemorrhage. J Intensive Care Med 2020;35(3):211–8.
25. Lazaridis C, Rusin CG, Robertson CS. Secondary brain injury: predicting and preventing insults. Neuropharmacology 2019;145(Pt B):145–52. https://doi.org/10.1016/j.neuropharm.2018.06.00.
26. Lefrant JY, Muller L, de La Coussaye JE, et al. Temperature measurement in intensive care patients: comparison of urinary bladder, oesophageal, rectal, axillary, and inguinal methods versus pulmonary artery core method. Intensive Care Med 2003;29(3):414–8.
27. Li Q, Zhang L-N, Tao X-M, et al. Temperature sensors: review of flexible temperature sensing networks for wearable physiological monitoring. Adv Healthc Mater 2017;6(12). https://doi.org/10.1002/adhm.201770059.
28. Kurashvili P, Olson D. Temperature management and nursing care of the patient with acute ischemic stroke. Stroke (1970) 2015;46(9):e205–7.
29. Jarrah S, Dziodzio J, Lord C, et al. Surface cooling after cardiac arrest: effectiveness, skin safety, and adverse events in routine clinical practice. Neurocrit Care 2011;14(3):382–8.
30. Soleimanpour H, Rahmani F, Golzari SE, et al. Main complications of mild induced hypothermia after cardiac arrest: a review article. J Cardiovasc Thorac Res 2014;6(1):1–8.
31. Prunet B, Lacroix G, Bordes J, et al. Catheter related venous thrombosis with cooling and warming catheters: two case reports. Cases J 2009;2(1):8857.
32. Jain A, Gray M, Slisz S, et al. Shivering treatments for targeted temperature management: a review. J Neurosci Nurs 2018;50(2):63–7.

33. Choi HA, Ko S-B, Presciutti M, et al. Prevention of shivering during therapeutic temperature modulation: the Columbia anti-shivering protocol. Neurocrit Care 2011;14(3):389–94.
34. Lavallée JF, Gray TA, Dumville J, et al. The effects of care bundles on patient outcomes: a systematic review and meta-analysis. Implementation Sci : IS 2017; 12(1):142.
35. Skaggs MKD, Daniels JF, Hodge AJ, et al. Using the evidence-based practice service nursing bundle to increase patient satisfaction. J Emerg Nurs 2018; 44(1):37–45.
36. Wang Y, Lim LL, Levi C, et al. Influence of admission body temperature on stroke mortality. Stroke 2000;31(2):404–9.
37. Powers WJ, Derdeyn CP, Biller J, et al. 2015 American Heart association/American stroke association focused update of the 2013 guidelines for the early management of patients with acute ischemic stroke regarding endovascular treatment: a guideline for healthcare professionals from the American Heart association/American stroke association. Stroke (1970) 2015;46(10):3020–35.
38. Greer DM, Funk SE, Reaven NL, et al. Impact of fever on outcome in patients with stroke and neurologic injury: a comprehensive meta-analysis. Stroke 2008; 39(11):3029–35.
39. Ringleb PA, Bousser MG, Ford G, et al. Guidelines for management of ischaemic stroke and transient ischaemic attack 2008. Cerebrovasc Dis (Basel, Switzerland) 2008;25(5):457–507.
40. Intercollegiate Stroke Working Party. National clinical guideline for stroke. 4th edition. London: Royal College of Physicians; 2012.
41. Ajčević M, Buoite Stella A, Furlanis G, et al. A novel non-invasive thermometer for continuous core body temperature: comparison with tympanic temperature in an acute stroke clinical setting. Sensors 2022;22(13). https://doi.org/10.3390/s22134760.
42. Nordberg P, Taccone FS, Castren M, et al. Design of the PRINCESS trial: prehospital resuscitation intra-nasal cooling effectiveness survival study (PRINCESS). BMC Emerg Med 2013;13:21.
43. Lipman GS, Eifling KP, Ellis MA, et al. Wilderness Medical Society practice guidelines for the prevention and treatment of heat-related illness: 2014 update. Wilderness Environ Med 2014;25(4 Suppl):S55–65.
44. Hong JM, Choi ES, Park SY. Selective brain cooling: a new horizon of neuroprotection. Front Neurol 2022;13:873165.
45. Badjatia N, Strongilis E, Gordon E, et al. Metabolic impact of shivering during therapeutic temperature modulation: the Bedside Shivering Assessment Scale. Stroke 2008;39(12):3242–7.

Stroke Risk Related to Coronavirus Disease-2019
What Have We Learned?

Pamela Pourciau, MSN, NP-C, SCRN, NC-BC*, Britta C. Smith, DNP, FNP-C

KEYWORDS

- Ischemic stroke • Risk • COVID-19 • SARS-CoV-2

KEY POINTS

- Coronavirus disease-2019 (COVID-19) and stroke risk.
- Stroke risk in severe acute respiratory syndrome coronavirus 2.
- Ischemic stroke in patients with COVID-19.

INTRODUCTION

Since its initial outbreak in December 2019, the novel severe acute respiratory syndrome coronavirus 2 (SARS-CoV-2) (coronavirus disease-2019 [COVID-19]) virus with its associated severe acute respiratory disease and pneumonia began to spread worldwide (**Fig. 1, Tables 1** and **2**).[1] Though COVID-19 is primarily associated with the pulmonary system, the virus can lead to damaging diseases that affect multiple organ systems including the central nervous system. Various neurologic manifestations and disorders associated with COVID-19 can range from mild symptoms such as headache or myalgias to more severe disorders including Guillain–Barre' syndrome, seizures, and psychosis. Though some of these neurologic associations are mild and likely reversible, significant numbers of patients with COVID-19 experience a stroke.[1]

On March 11, 2020, the World Health Organization declared COVID-19 to be a pandemic and since then, reports of increased risk for acute ischemic stroke (AIS) in those with COVID-19 began to emerge and continue to evolve.[2]

DISCUSSION

Stroke care is based on the American Stroke Association Guidelines.[3,4] Timely presentation to the nearest hospital reduces the delay of care to potentially offer

East Jefferson Neurological Associates, 3800 Houma Boulevard, Suite 325, Metairie, LA 70006, USA
* Corresponding author.
E-mail address: pamela.pourciau@lcmchealth.org

Crit Care Nurs Clin N Am 35 (2023) 53–65
https://doi.org/10.1016/j.cnc.2022.10.001
ccnursing.theclinics.com
0899-5885/23/© 2022 Elsevier Inc. All rights reserved.

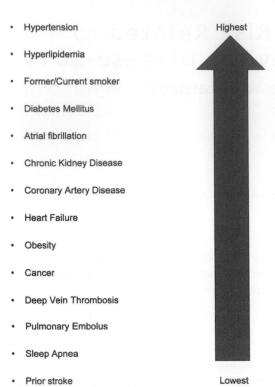

- Hypertension
- Hyperlipidemia
- Former/Current smoker
- Diabetes Mellitus
- Atrial fibrillation
- Chronic Kidney Disease
- Coronary Artery Disease
- Heart Failure
- Obesity
- Cancer
- Deep Vein Thrombosis
- Pulmonary Embolus
- Sleep Apnea
- Prior stroke

Highest

Lowest

Fig. 1. Vascular risk factor prevalence in patients.[32]

interventions such as intravenous thrombolytic or cerebral thrombectomy. Delay of care increases the likelihood of being ineligible for these interventions, thereby increasing mortality and morbidity related to stroke. The COVID-19 pandemic caused a tremendous stain on the health care system worldwide because of the lack of treatment methods for patients infected with COVID-19. It overburdened emergency rooms and overwhelmed medical staff which impacted stroke care. Patients with transient ischemic attacks or those with mild stroke symptoms refrained from presenting to the emergency room or declined admission out of fear.[5]

At the beginning of the pandemic, The World Health Organization had recommended the reduction of exposure with the use of protective personal equipment, social distancing, avoiding crowds, home confinement, and for health care systems to cease all nonessential services and elective surgeries to reduce the spread of the virus.[6] Studies suggested that because of the isolation requirements, people with stroke symptoms either did not know they were experiencing a stroke or delayed seeking care thereby limiting interventions.[5]

Research

Early in the pandemic, COVID-19 began to become associated with AIS. Patients with the COVID-19 infection in China were noted with coagulopathy and antiphospholipid antibodies. They were elderly patients with severe infection prone to cerebrovascular events and younger patients, less than 50 years of age with large vessel strokes.[7] A study in the United States confirmed a significant incident of acute stroke in patients with COVID-19 infection and found COVID-19 to be an independent risk factor for AIS. Therefore, patients with COVID-19 should have continuous monitoring for AIS.[8]

Table 1
Correlation of cerebrovascular disease with coronavirus disease-2019

Study Methodology	Neurologic Manifestations	Total Number	Number of Strokes	%	Authors
Retrospective observational	Cerebrovascular disease Ischemic stroke – 5 Hemorrhagic stroke – 1	214	6	2.8	Mao et al,[10] 2020
Single-center retrospective, observational	Cerebrovascular disease Ischemic stroke – 10 Hemorrhagic stroke – 1	219	11	5	Li et al,[13] 2020
Multicenter, multinational, observational, systematic review, meta-analysis	Strokes Ischemic stroke – 123 Hemorrhagic stroke – 27 Cerebral venous thrombosis – 6	17,779	156	0.9 (Pooled risk)	Shahjouei et al,[14] 2020
Systematic review, meta-analysis	Ischemic stroke	8577	226	2.6	Huth et al,[15] 2021
Multicenter, retrospective	Ischemic stroke	41,971	1143	2.7	Srivastava et al,[16] 2021
Multicenter, retrospective	Ischemic stroke Hemorrhagic stroke Cerebral venous thrombosis	725	34 6 2	4.7 0.8 0.3	Mahedmmedi et al,[17] 2020
Retrospective, observational	Ischemic stroke Hemorrhagic stroke	841	11	1.3	Romero-Sanchez et al,[18] 2020
Systematic review, meta-analysis	Acute cerebrovascular disease Acute ischemic stroke—1329 Intracerebral hemorrhage—180	108,571	1409	1.3	Nanooni et al,[19] 2021

(continued on next page)

Table 1
(continued)

Study Methodology	Neurologic Manifestations	Total Number	Number of Strokes	%	Authors
Retrospective cohort	Acute cerebrovascular disease Acute ischemic stroke/TIA—160 Intracerebral hemorrhage—44 Subarachnoid hemorrhage—33 Epidural/subdural hemorrhage—21 Central venous thromboses—2 Not otherwise classified—24	21, 073	284	1.4 (Pooled risk)	Shakil et al,[20] 2022
Retrospective cohort	Acute ischemic stroke	8163	103	1.6	Qureshi et al,[21] 2021
Retrospective observational cohort	Ischemic stroke	14,483	156	0.8	Siegler,[22] 2021

Table 2
Features of stroke in coronavirus disease-2019

Common Findings Across Studies Reviewed	References
More common in younger patients (mean < 55 years) without classic vascular risk factors	Shahjouei et al,[24] 2021; Jabbour et al,[25] 2022; Zhang et al,[7] 2020
More common among younger (ages 65 to 74 years) Medicare beneficiaries and among Medicare beneficiaries without prior history of stroke.	Yang et al,[26] 2022
Higher prevalence of cryptogenic stroke	Shahjouei et al,[24] 2021; Yang et al,[26] 2022; Stein et al,[27] 2021; Siegler et al,[22] 2021
Increased incidence of large vessel occlusion stroke	Lee et al,[28] 2020; John et al,[29] 2020; Shahjouei et al,[24] 2021 Shahjouei et al,[30] 2021; Roman et al,[23] Li et al,[13] 2020; Nanonni,[19] 2021
Smaller incidence of small vessel occlusion stroke and lacunar stroke	Shahjouei et al,[24] 2021
Stroke more severe	Ntaios,[31] 2020
Patients more critically ill, on mechanical ventilator, with ischemic heart disease	Li et al,[10] 2020
Higher mortality (in-hospital)	Nanonni et al,[19] 2021; Quereshi,[21] 2021; Siegler,[22] 2021
Increased morbidity and mortality	Stein et al,[27] 2021; Ntaios,[31] 2020; Jabbour et al,[25] 2022
Worse functional outcomes	Ntaios,[31] 2020
Increased incidence of stroke with severe COVID-19	Mao et al,[10] 2020; Nanonni et al,[19] 2021
Increased incidence of multi-territory strokes	Nanonni et al,[19] 2021; Yang et al,[26] 2022

Reports of neurologic involvement in 30% to 50% of all individuals with SARS-CoV-2 infection have been defined, with almost half of these attributable to stroke.[9] According to Mao and associates, early reports from Wuhan ascertained that more than 36% of patients with COVID-19 had some degree of neurologic involvement, most commonly affecting the central nervous system.[10] Maury and colleagues[11] found that up to 73% of hospitalized patients with COVID-19 experienced some type of neurologic symptom. These same authors also reported that acute cerebrovascular diseases, predominately AIS, have been found in 0.7% to 5.8% of hospitalized patients with COVID-19. The increased risk of ischemic stroke and intracranial hemorrhage with or post-COVID-19 was evident in study after study. An alarming finding by Taquet and colleagues[12] showed that the incidence of ischemic stroke was almost one in 10 or (three in 100 for a first stroke) in patients with encephalopathy ($n = 236$, 379).

In one of the earliest studies, with data collected from January 16, 2020, to February 19, 2020, from three special care centers in Wuhan, China, Mao and colleagues[10] found that of the 214 patients, 36.4% or 78 patients had neurologic sequelae. Severe infection, characterized by respiratory status, was seen in 88 patients (41.1%) and of those, 5.7% had an acute cerebrovascular disease and 14.8% showed impairment of consciousness. Those with severe infection were older and had more comorbidities, specifically hypertension.[10]

A review of 11 studies outlines the frequency that cerebrovascular disease is shown to correlate with COVID-19, with the focus being ischemic stroke.

Roman and colleagues[23] found that central nervous system manifestations such as headache, partial or total loss of smell (hyposmia, anosmia) and distorted (dysgeusia), diminished (hypogeusia), or loss (ageusia) of taste perception to be common early symptoms of COVID-19 infection. In fact, changes in taste and smell sensation were often used as primary screening symptoms for COVID-19. Considering the anatomy of the olfactory nerve and cribriform plate, this might suggest how the virus gains access to the brain. Respiratory failure is often the main cause of death related to COVID-19 and this pathway may explain how the COVID-19 virus gains access to the rhinencephalon and brainstem centers.[23]

Cerebrovascular disease, primarily large vessel ischemic strokes, and to a lesser degree cerebral venous thrombosis, intracerebral hemorrhage, and subarachnoid hemorrhage, are thought to occur as part of a thrombotic state generated by the virus attaching to ACE2 endothelial receptors leading to extensive endothelial inflammation, coagulopathy, as well as arterial and venous thromboses.[23]

Below is a table of common stroke features obtained from a variety of research studies primarily, from data procured in 2019 - early 2021.

Yang and colleagues[26] in their systematic review and meta-analysis of Medicare beneficiaries 65 years and older, examined the characteristics and outcomes of patients with COVID-19 and stroke and found a pooled incidence of 1.4% of acute cerebrovascular disease. In their study, they found that most patients admitted with COVID-19 symptoms developed stroke a few days later. The strokes were usually ischemic in nature, cryptogenic in cause, and often distinguished by multiple cerebral infarctions.[26]

When determining risk factors for stroke incidence in patients with COVID-19, Nannoni and associates[19] examined four studies. These researchers were able to compare clinical characteristics of patients with both COVID-19 and cerebrovascular disease ($n = 113$) and those without cerebrovascular disease ($n = 11,683$). Patients with COVID-19 who also had cerebrovascular risk factors such as hypertension, diabetes mellitus, and coronary artery disease showed an increased risk for stroke. The patients were also older and there were no differences in male versus female. Interestingly, their research did not show any significant difference between smokers and nonsmokers.[19]

In their meta-analysis of clinical characteristics of patients with both COVID-19 and acute cerebrovascular disease, the above authors[19] examined 50 studies. The authors found that median age was 65.3 years with the majority being male. Hypertension, diabetes mellitus, and dyslipidemia were the most common vascular risk factors. Severe COVID-19 was seen in 61% of the patients with 86.7% demonstrating radiologic evidence of pneumonia and 14.8% of patients were afflicted with pulmonary embolism.[19]

Clinical implications for the above study[19] include:

- Incidence of stroke could complicate the course of COVID-19 with those older and having more severe infection presenting a higher risk
- Though incidence of stroke in COVID-19 population was less than 2%, this would have a global impact because of sheer numbers of people infected by the virus
- Clinicians, including nurses, should be vigilant in their bedside assessments observing for acute neurologic symptom development in patients with COVID-19
- Patients who are intubated and/or sedated require close monitoring incorporating assessment of pupillary reactivity and utilization of the Glasgow Coma Scale which might render discovery of abnormal neurologic manifestations

- Patients who have abnormal coagulation studies or other thrombotic complications deserve close observation for development of sudden abnormal neurologic dysfunction
- Providers should follow a protected stroke pathway for patients with stroke presentation who also have suspected or confirmed COVID-19 infection.

Another study by Qureshi and peers found that in patients with COVID-19, the proportion of patients with hypertension, diabetes mellitus, hyperlipidemia, atrial fibrillation, and congestive heart failure was significantly higher among those with AIS.[21]

Xu and colleagues[32] in 2021 found some similarities in risk factor prevalence, specifically with hypertension, hyperlipidemia, diabetes mellitus, atrial fibrillation, and heart failure, in their study as outlined below:

- Hypertension highest
- Hyperlipidemia
- Former/current smoker
- Diabetes mellitus
- Atrial fibrillation
- Chronic kidney disease
- Coronary artery disease
- Heart failure
- Obesity
- Cancer
- Deep vein thrombosis
- Pulmonary embolus
- Sleep apnea
- Prior stroke lowest

In an international multicenter retrospective study including 50 comprehensive stroke centers with a cohort of 575 patients with large vessel occlusion, Jabbour and colleagues[25] found that 194 of the patients were positive for COVID-19. The group members were younger (62.5 years), had fewer risk factors for cerebrovascular disease, and experienced higher morbidity and mortality rates.

Mechanisms of Hypercoagulability in Coronavirus Disease-2019

The specific process through which COVID-19 lends to a hypercoagulable state in the infected population is unknown but understanding the pathophysiology of the hypercoagulable state is key to optimizing treatment to those with COVID-19-induced ischemic stroke and for the prevention of ischemic stroke in those with COVID-19 infection. Inflammation and hypercoagulability are influenced by a cytokine storm that interacts with the coagulation cascade. Studies show cytokines cause neutrophil extracellular traps (NETs), which turn on the extrinsic and intrinsic coagulation pathways creating thrombin that promotes coagulation and leads to AIS.[33]

COVID-19 invades endothelial cells in vessels, tissues, and organs through the angiotensin-converting enzyme 2 (ACE 2), which can damage renal, intestine, and lung tissue. It is a known fact that damaged endothelial cells are related to ischemic stroke. Interestingly, cerebral neurons and vascular smooth muscle cells have the ACE 2 receptor that allows the virus to cross the blood–brain barrier creating central nervous system damage and promote central thrombosis.[33]

Patients with severe cases of COVID-19 have low platelet and lymphocyte counts and increased neutrophils, D-dimer and C-reactive protein levels. It has been hypothesized the virus interferes with lymphocytes by decreasing platelet production, increasing platelet destruction, and then possibly to thrombosis leading to platelet consumption. Platelet activation related to a hypercoagulable state in patients with COVID-19 may increase the risk of AIS.[33]

During the inflammatory cascade, neutrophils use NETs to capture bacteria. These NETs are made from DNA and proteins which are possibly related to diseases in a hypercoagulable state promoting thrombosis, which in turn may contribute to AIS.[33]

Activated platelet release particles (MPs) result from apoptosis of cells. They are the result of various cells such as erythrocytes, platelets, and endothelial cells. MPs are suspected to cause hypercoagulability in many disease states including stroke.[33]

The immune system uses the complement system for protection against viruses. Lack of an adequately functional complement system can cause a system wide inflammatory response creating tissue damage. Coagulation and micro-thrombosis are also associated with the activation of the complement system.[33]

Patients who become hypoxic from the development of acute respiratory distress syndrome with severe COVID-19 infection trigger pathways leading to thrombosis. It is suspected that bacteria or viruses promote antiphospholipid antibodies thereby patients with COVID-19 promoting antiphospholipid production are at risk for hypercoagulability state-induced ischemic stroke.[33]

MBonde and colleagues[9] proposed the pathophysiology of AIS with. COVID-19 involves:

- Inflammatory response
- Coagulopathy
- Endothelial dysfunction
- Platelet activation
- Cardioembolic phenomenon

Implications for Future Research

COVID-19 vaccination status is one cohort for new researchers to consider when collecting data and looking at the relationship between COVID-19 and stroke risk. Kakovan and associates indicate that vaccine-induced thrombotic thrombocytopenai (VITT) may be associated with stroke post-COVID-19 vaccine.[34] Clinicians should be aware of possible stroke after COVID-19 vaccination to ensure rapid diagnosis and treatment. Should a patient develop any new neurologic symptoms, especially constant headaches, within a month of receiving a COVID-19 vaccine, moderate suspicion for stroke should be considered. Laboratory testing for possible VITT could include platelet count, D-dimer, anti-PF4 antibody, fibrinogen level, and brain imaging. In addition, those with VITT should be evaluated for concurrent thrombotic diagnoses such as deep vein thrombosis, pulmonary thromboembolism, and venous thrombosis.[34]

Stroke and cerebral venous thrombosis have been reported in the Vaccine Adverse Event Reporting System (VAERS) specific to the Pfizer-BioNTech, Moderna, and J&J/Janssen COVID-19 vaccines.[16] Though there is not yet a plethora of data supporting this, consideration of COVID-19 vaccine status is not unreasonable.

Huth and colleagues[15] concluded that more robust studies using standardized screening and case definitions are warranted. This was certainly apparent with our literature review and review of studies.

In their retrospective study ($n = 368$), Oates and associates[35] found support for the use of transthoracic echocardiography (TTE) in patients with COVID-19 to assist in risk detection of ischemic stroke. The authors developed a composite risk score using clinical and echocardiographic characteristics:

- Age less than 55 years
- Systolic blood pressure greater than 140 mm Hg
- Anticoagulation before admission
- Left atrial dilation
- Left ventricular thrombus

The researchers[35] found an increased incidence of left atrial dilation and left ventricular thrombus (48.3% vs 27.9%, P = .04:4.2% vs 0.7%, P = .03) in patients with ischemic stroke. TTE is currently used as a part of the diagnostic workup for stroke and TIA. This non-invasive diagnostic test could be used more in those with severe COVID-19 with suspected stroke.[35]

CLINICS CARE POINTS

- Worldwide research examining comparisons of coronavirus disease-2019 (COVID-19) positive and COVID-19 negative stroke cohorts show a relationship between COVID-19 and ischemic stroke.

- Providers must address control of risk factors such as hypertension, high coagulability states, and diabetes mellitus in patients with COVID-19.

- Public health campaigns focusing on stroke recognition and emphasizing the need to seek care for stroke, even during a pandemic, are needed.

- COVID-19 best practice guidelines should be incorporated within the American Heart Association/America Stroke Association Stroke guidelines.

- COVID-19-associated stroke can affect the young, with or without cerebrovascular risk factors.

- Morbidity and mortality are much worse in patients with COVID-19 and stroke as compared with patients with only stroke

- Hypercoagulability studies should be considered and completed on younger patients with stroke, with or without COVID-19 symptoms

- On patients with suspected stroke, a full stroke workup is warranted, even if done post-discharge through an outpatient setting

- More robust research is needed for the prevention and treatment of COVID-19

Clinical Relevance

In summary, there are many elements that participate in the activation of the immune system in patients infected with COVID-19 leading to a hypercoagulable state beginning with the trigger of a cytokine storm that creates subsequent endothelial cell damage and the production of NETs, distribution of MPs, platelet activation, and the initiation of the complement system. It is also important to understand hypoxia is a causal factor in COVID-19-related stroke. The cerebrum is sensitive to changes in oxygenation, so hypoxia can not only cause interstitial cerebral edema but also initiate the coagulation cascade.[33]

Antithrombotic therapy targeting the various mechanisms that lead to thrombosis should be considered in COVID-19-infected patients. Antithrombotic therapy increases oxygen saturation levels in the blood and the coagulopathy. Complications of COVID-19 lead to increased risk for AIS. Therefore, anticoagulation should be initiated early during the initial phase of COVID-19 to prevent AIS.[33]

Since the pandemic, studies have alluded to stoke patients with COVID-19 being younger and having a higher initial admission National Institutes of Health Stroke Scale (NIHSS) than those without COVID-19 infection. Laboratory data to assess for hyper-coagulation or inflammation such as d-dimer, interleukin-6, C-reactive protein, fibrinogen, and platelets are usually elevated in the COVID-19 patient. All efforts should be made to adhere to national guidelines for stroke care.[36]

The COVID-19 pandemic created a greater opportunity for telemedicine. Utilization of telemedicine enabled social distancing and the ability to maintain isolation between patients and providers. Tele-Neurology is available to allow vascular neurologists to oversee stoke activations in remote facilities or where expertise is unavailable. It also provides quick use of the NIHSS to provide an assessment from symptom onset to treatment and management more efficiently.[37]

Patient evaluation for symptoms of an ischemic stroke should result in a full stroke workup. Typically, an initial neurologic evaluation is performed to assess deficits followed by cerebral and vascular imaging is performed. A cardiac workup and coagulation panel are included. Results of the imaging and patient eligibility as per stroke guidelines[3,4] determine interventions of intravenous thrombolytic or mechanical thrombectomy.[37]

Clinicians may assume stroke symptoms typically occur in the elderly population, but what we have seen since the COVID-19 pandemic are younger people including children experiencing stroke symptoms.[37,38] Stroke in the young usually includes further workup to explain their hypercoagulable state or cause for stroke. It is important for nursing to use a standardized tool such as the NIHSS to monitor for subtle neurologic changes in patients which may not be otherwise explained and advocating for neuroimaging. A standardized inpatient stroke code protocol should be implemented and familiar. As clinicians, identifying patient risk factors for stroke and being able to identify neurologic changes early, and knowing the time when the patient was last known normal are essential for timely stroke intervention.[39]

SUMMARY

In January 2022, for the 20th year in a row, nurses were ranked number one as the most trusted profession[40] despite the pandemic and its related critical staffing and equipment shortages, threat to their personal safety and that of their patients, co-workers, and families, and extreme physical and mental duress. Data and quality of care have long been linked to promote optimum patient outcomes. Accuracy of that data is crucial. As nurses are the largest group of health care professionals and play a key role in patient safety and quality outcomes, it is imperative that they have access to quality, robust data and be knowledgeable about its interpretation so that they can make informed practice decisions.[41]

Three years into the COVID-19 pandemic, there is growing evidence that the increased incidence of vascular risk factors with concomitant proinflammatory and procoagulation biomarkers show a distinct relationship of ischemic stroke risk in patients with SARS-CoV-2 infection.[7] Despite governmental assurances that the pandemic is over, long-term effects of COVID-19 continue to evolve. Other than vaccination, academic literature is still lacking with respect to prevention and early treatment of COVID-19 as well its long-term effects.

DISCLOSURE

The authors have nothing to disclose.

REFERENCES

1. Katsanos AH, Palaiodimou L, Zand R, et al. The impact of SARS-CoV-2 on stroke epidemiology and care: a meta-analysis. Ann Neurol 2021;89(2):380–8. https://doi.org/10.1002/ana.25967.

2. Finsterer Josef, Scorza FA, Scorza CA, et al. Ischemic stroke in 455 COVID-19 patients. Clinics 2022;77. https://doi.org/10.1016/j.clinsp.2022.100012.

3. Powers WJ, Rabinstein AA, Ackerson T, et al. Guidelines for the early management of patients with acute ischemic stroke: 2019 update to the 2018 guidelines for the early management of acute ischemic stroke: a guideline for health care professionals from the american heart association/american stroke association. Stroke 2019;50(12):e344–418 [published correction appears in stroke. 2019;50(12):e440-e441].

4. Kernan WN, Ovbiagele B, Black HR, et al. Guidelines for the prevention of stroke in patients with stroke and transient ischemic attack: a guideline for health care professionals from the American Heart Association/American Stroke Association. Stroke 2014;45(7):2160–2236 [published correction appears in Stroke. 2015;46(2):e54].

5. Schlachetzki F, Theek C, Hubert ND, et al. Low stroke incidence in the TEMPiS telestroke network during COVID-19 pandemic: effect of lockdown on thrombolysis and thrombectomy. J Telemed Telecare 2020;28(7):481–7.

6. World Health Organization. Coronavirus disease (COVID-19) pandemic. World health organization; 2022. Retrieved August 7, 2022, from. https://www.who.int/emergencies/disease/novel-coronavirus-2019.

7. Zhang Y, Xiao M, Zhang S, et al. Coagulopathy and antiphospholipid antibodies in patients with COVID-19. N Engl J Med 2020;382(38):1.

8. Belani P, Schefflein J, Kihira S, et al. COVID-19 is an independent risk factor for acute ischemic stroke. Am J Neuroradiology 2020;41(8):1361–4.

9. Mbonde AA, O'Carroll CB, Grill MF, et al. Stroke features, risk factors, and pathophysiology in SARS-CoV-2-infected patients. Mayo Clin Proc Innov Qual Outcomes 2022;6(2):156–65.

10. Mao L, Jin H, Wang M. Neurologic manifestations of hospitalized patients with coronavirus disease 2019 in wuhan, China. JAMA Neurol 2020;77(6):683–90.

11. Maury A, Lyoubi A, Peiffer-Smadja N, et al. Neurological manifestations associated with SARS-CoV-2 and other coronaviruses: a narrative review for clinicians. Rev Neurol (Paris) 2021;177(1–2):51–64.

12. Taquet M, Geddes J, Husain M, et al. 6-month neurological and psychiatric outcomes in 236379 survivors of COVID-19: a retrospective cohort study using electronic health records. Lancet Psychiatry 2021;8:416–22.

13. Li Y, Li M, Wang M, et al. Acute cerebrovascular disease following COVID-19: a single center, retrospective, observational study. Stroke Vasc Neurol 2020;5(3):279–84.

14. Shahjouei S, Naderi S, Li J, et al. Risk of stroke in hospitalized SARS-CoV-2 infected patients: a multinational study. EBioMedicine 2020;59:102939.

15. Huth SF, Cho SM, Robba C, et al. Neurological manifestations of coronavirus disease 2019: a comprehensive review and meta-analysis of the first 6 months of pandemic reporting. Front Neurol 2021;12:664599.

16. Srivastava PK, Zhang S, Xian Y, et al. Acute ischemic stroke in patients with COVID-19: an analysis from get with the guidelines-stroke. Stroke 2021;52(5):1826–9.

17. Mahammedi A, Saba L, Vagal A, et al. Imaging of neurologic disease in hospitalized patients with COVID-19: an Italian multicenter retrospective observational study. Radiology 2020;297(2):E270–3.
18. Romero-Sánchez CM, Díaz-Maroto I, Fernández-Díaz E. Neurologic manifestations in hospitalized patients with COVID-19: the ALBACOVID registry. Neurology 2020;95(8):e1060–70.
19. Nannoni S, de Groot R, Bell S, et al. Stroke in COVID-19: a systematic review and meta-analysis. Int J Stroke 2021;16(2):137–49.
20. Shakil SS, Emmons-Bell S, Rutan C, et al. Stroke among patients hospitalized with Covid-19: results from the american heart association COVID-19 cardiovascular disease registry. Stroke 2022;53(3):800–7.
21. Qureshi AI, Baskett WI, Huang W, et al. Acute ischemic stroke and COVID-19: an analysis of 27 676 patients. Stroke 2021;52(3):905–12.
22. Siegler JE, Cardona P, Arenillas JF, et al. Cerebrovascular events and outcomes in hospitalized patients with COVID-19: the SVIN COVID-19 multinational registry. Int J Stroke 2021;16(4):437–47.
23. Román GC, Spencer PS, Reis J, et al. The neurology of COVID-19 revisited: a proposal from the environmental neurology specialty group of the world federation of neurology to implement international neurological registries. J Neurol Sci 2020;414:116884. Available at: https://www.ncbi.nlm.nih.gov/pmc/articles/PMC7204734/.
24. Shahjouei S, Tsivgoulis G, Farahmand G, et al. SARS-CoV-2 and stroke characteristics: a report from the multinational COVID-19 stroke study group. Stroke 2021;52(5):e117–30.
25. Jabbour P, Dmytriw AA, Sweid A, et al. Characteristics of a COVID-19 cohort with large vessel occlusion: a multicenter international study. Neurosurgery 2022; 90(6):725–33.
26. Yang Q, Tong X, George MG, et al. COVID-19 and risk of acute ischemic stroke among medicare beneficiaries aged 65 years or older: self-controlled case series study. Neurology 2022;98(8):e778–89.
27. Stein LK, Mayman NA, Dhamoon MS, et al. The emerging association between COVID-19 and acute stroke. Trends Neurosci 2021;44(Issue 7):527–37.
28. Lee KW, Yusof Khan AHK, Ching SM, et al. Stroke and novel coronavirus infection in humans: a systematic review and meta-analysis. Front Neurol 2020;11:1196.
29. John S, Kesav P, Mifsud VA, et al. Characteristics of large-vessel occlusion associated with COVID-19 and ischemic stroke. Am J Neuroradiol 2020;41:2263–8.
30. Shahjouei S, Anyaehie M, Koza E, et al. SARS-CoV-2 is a culprit for some, but not all acute ischemic strokes: a report from the multinational COVID-19 stroke study group. J Clin Med 2021;10(5):931.
31. Ntaios G, Michel P, Georgiopoulos G, et al. Characteristics and outcomes in patients with COVID-19 and acute ischemic stroke: the global COVID-19 stroke registry. Stroke 2020;51(9):e254–8 (00392499),.
32. Xu Y, Zhuang Y, Kang L. A review of neurological involvement in patients with SARS-CoV-2 infection. Med Sci Monit 2021;27:e932962.
33. Abou-Ismail MY, Diamond A, Kapoor S, et al. The hypercoagulable state in COVID-19: incidence, pathophysiology, and management. Thromb Res 2020; 194:101–15.
34. Kakovan M, Ghorbani Shirkouhi S, Zarei M, et al. Stroke associated with COVID-19 vaccines. J Stroke Cerebrovasc Dis 2022;31(6):106440.
35. Oates Connor P, et al. Using clinical and echocardiographic characteristics to characterize the risk of ischemic stroke in patients with COVID-19. J Stroke

Cerebrovasc Dis 2022;31(2). N.PAG. EBSCOhost, Available at: https://doi-org. ezproxy.nicholls.edu/10.1016/j.jstrokecerebrovasdis.2021.106217.

36. Qi X, Keith KA, Huang JH. COVID-19 and stroke: a review. Brain Hemorrhages 2021;2(2):76–83. Epub 2020 Nov 17. PMID: 33225251; PMCID: PMC7670261.

37. Appavu B, Deng D, Dowling MM, et al. Arteritis and large vessel occlusive strokes in children after COVID-19 infection. Pediatrics 2021;147(3):1–7.

38. Coronado Munoz A, Tasayco J, Morales W, et al. High incidence of stroke and mortality in pediatric critical care patients with COVID-19 in Peru. Pediatr Res 2022;91:1730–4.

39. Assuncao C, Evers B, Martins C, et al. Comparison of code stroke response times between emergency department and inpatient settings in a primary stroke center. J Neurol Res 2021;11. Available at: https://www.neurores.org/index.php/ neurores/article/view/6888/658.

40. Saad L. Military brass, judges among professions at new image lows. 2022. Retrieved from. https://news.gallup.com/poll/388649/military-brass-judges-among-professions-new-image-lows.aspx.

41. Glasman KS. Using data in nursing practice. 2017. Retrieved from. https://www. myamericannurse.com/wp-content/uploads/2017/11/ant11-Data-1030.pdf.

Decompressive Hemicraniectomy in the Stroke Patient

Carey Heck, PhD, CRNP, AGACNP-BC, CNRN

KEYWORDS

- Neurosurgery • Decompression hemicraniectomy • Stroke • Outcomes

KEY POINTS

- Decompressive hemicraniectomy (DHC) is a life-saving procedure to relieve intracranial hypertension.
- Severe disability following DHC is not uncommon, particularly in older patients.
- Complications following DHC are significant and require acute monitoring.
- Goals of care discussions before consideration of DHC are important to ascertain patient/family understanding and acceptance of unfavorable outcomes.
- Socioeconomic factors adversely affect access to comprehensive stroke care, including DHC.

BACKGROUND

Globally, a new stroke occurs every 3 seconds resulting in 12.2 million new strokes annually. Stroke is the second leading cause of death globally and accounts for an estimated $861 billion in associated costs. The lifetime risk of stroke has increased by 50% over the last 20 years presenting challenges for health care systems to deliver quality, cost-effective care.[1,2] Treatment of strokes includes both medical and surgical care. One such surgical procedure, a decompressive hemicraniectomy (DHC), is performed to improve cerebral blood flow and decrease intracranial hypertension as a result of cerebral edema.[3–5] The procedure, which involves removal of a large portion of the skull to reduce cerebral edema, has been shown to decrease mortality but is also associated with an increase in severe disability in patients who survive.[6–10] An understanding of DHC in stroke care and the management of patients post-procedure is essential to provide optimal patient outcomes.

The historical foundation of DHC, as well as the risks, benefits, and complications, is well-documented in the extant literature.[11–14] The precedent of DHC as an intervention

Adult-Gerontology Acute Care Nurse Practitioner Program, Thomas Jefferson University, 901 Walnut Street, Suite 815, Philadelphia, PA 19107, USA
E-mail address: Carey.Heck@Jefferson.edu

Crit Care Nurs Clin N Am 35 (2023) 67–81
https://doi.org/10.1016/j.cnc.2022.10.004
ccnursing.theclinics.com

to reduce intracranial hypertension is found in the procedure known as trephination. Evidence of trephination, or the creation of an opening into a skull to drain fluid or remove lesions, has been found in skulls as early as the Paleolithic era.[12,13] Prehistoric skulls bearing evidence of trephination have been found across the globe and point to widespread usage and the procedure's acceptance as an option for a variety of ailments. Trephined skulls with evidence of cranial injury suggest the purpose of trephination in early history was as a treatment of traumatic brain injuries. Not all skulls bore evidence of injury, which has led to speculation that the procedure was performed for reasons less well defined by science such as spiritual, magical, or ritualistic purposes.[11,12] Indications for trephination are found in the ancient writings of Hippocrates as an intervention for skull fractures.[14] Modern trephination and by extension craniotomy continues to be used in the management of cerebral edema, most frequently in traumatic brain injury (TBI) and large middle cerebral artery (MCA) strokes.

A robust body of literature exists describing DHC in TBI.[14–17] The Decompressive Craniectomy[16] and Randomized Evaluation of Surgery with Craniectomy for Uncontrollable Elevation of Intracranial Pressure[17] trials investigated the use of DHC in TBI patients. A decrease in mortality was clearly demonstrated in both studies. However, poor functional outcomes, defined as a modified Rankin Score (mRS) greater than 4, were prevalent in surviving patients.[16,17] The controversy associated with DHC is the clear survival benefit seen in patients undergoing DHC but who are then left with a dependent functional status.

The use of DHC for large MCA strokes has been extensively examined. Most notable are the European randomized controlled studies: the Decompressive Surgery for the Treatment of Malignant Infarction of the Middle Cerebral Artery (DESTINY) 6, Decompressive Craniectomy in Malignant Middle Cerebral Artery infarction 7, and the Hemicraniectomy After Middle Cerebral Artery infarction with Life-threatening Edema Trial.[8] These trials demonstrated a mortality reduction of 40% to 50% in patients with malignant cerebral edema (MCE) due to ischemic stroke but also demonstrated severe disability in surviving patients.[6–8] None of the studies demonstrated a significant reduction in disability as defined by an mRS of 0 to 3 at 6 months post-procedure.[9,10,18] Increased disability and poor functional outcomes were notable in patients over the age of 60 years who underwent DHC.[11]

The significance of surgical timing has been explored in the literature with inconclusive recommendations.[10,19,20] Back and colleagues[10] found an increase in poor functional outcomes associated with patients who underwent the procedure after 48 hours. Conversely, Garcia-Estrada and colleagues[19] found no difference in survival or favorable functional outcomes in patients undergoing DHC less than 48 hours or ≥48 hours. Despite controversy, DHC continues to be an important procedure for relieving intracranial pressure and reducing mortality in select patients.

The mortality and morbidity associated with DHC is not insignificant. The historically high mortality rates associated with the procedure led to skepticism that long-term survival was possible. Prehistoric skulls found at archaeological sites around the world bear evidence of trephination with bone changes suggesting patient survival after the procedure.[12] When first introduced to the medical community in the twentieth century, physicians and scientists dismissed the possibility of patient survival in light of the complications associated with the procedure.[12] Despite the high mortality rate, often due to infection in an era without the benefit of antibiotics, early modern trials demonstrated the benefits of trephination in the setting of cranial trauma. Subsequently, DHC was touted in the medical literature as a viable option for patients with increased cerebral edema.[11,12] As an understanding of brain pathophysiology increased along with advances in neurosurgical procedures, so too did the utilization of DHC. Kocher recommended that all cases of intracranial hypertension should be relieved by surgical trepanation. Initially used primarily in the TBI population, expansion to other patient populations occurred. Current guidelines have evolved from utilization of DHC in all cases of intracranial hypertension to a closer attention to patient selection, timing, alternative treatments, and patient outcomes.[21] These factors are essential to examine before any decision to perform a DHC.[22]

STATISTICS

Ischemic stroke accounts for 62% of all strokes with the majority occurring in patients aged 70 years or less. Although the incidence of stroke in the elderly has decreased, epidemiological studies have identified an increase in stroke among young adults aged 18 to 50 years.[2] In 2019, 11% of strokes occurred in young adults and 61% of strokes occurred in patients less than 70 years of age[1] The financial cost of stroke is significant with an estimated $861 billion in associated care.[1] Treatment goals in the management of stroke include a return to baseline function and prevention of secondary ischemia. Access to comprehensive, effective, and timely treatment modalities used in the management of ischemic stroke facilitate attainment of these goals. Standard management options include thrombolysis and reperfusion therapy. Thrombolysis within the 4.5 hour recommended time frame is the mainstay of therapy.[21] Other interventions, including endovascular therapy and surgical decompression, are of additional benefit to select patient groups.[15,21]

Even with standard management, a percentage of ischemic stroke patients will develop life-threatening complications requiring complex treatments to reduce mortality and preserve functional status. MCE represents an acute complication in patients with MCA strokes. MCE is characterized by extensive cerebral edema and neurological deterioration resulting in death or poor functional outcome. Up to 10% of patients with anterior circulation stroke and up to 40% of cerebellar strokes will develop MCE. Without intervention, the risk of death due to MCE is as high as 80%.[11,21,23] The risk of MCE is substantially reduced when thrombolytic therapy and recanalization procedures are used.[24,25] In patients with unilateral MCA infarctions, current recommendations support maximal medical therapy. Despite reperfusion therapy, neurological deterioration may still occur. For select patients experiencing progressive neurological deterioration, DHC is an option.

DECOMPRESSIVE CRANIOTOMY

DHC is a neurosurgical procedure categorized as primary or secondary. Primary DHC is an emergent, acute, life-saving procedure that reduces patient mortality but is associated with a higher incidence of complications. Secondary DHC is performed when other efforts to reduce intracranial hypertension have failed.[26,27] Surgical technique, technical improvements, and infection control measures have evolved over time and with-it improved patient outcomes. Current guidelines recommend DHC within 48 hours of symptom onset in patients with neurological deterioration due to cerebral edema despite medical therapy.[21]

When DHC is indicated, the procedure involves the creation of a large opening in the skull designed to reduce cerebral edema is performed. A frontal-temporal-parietal approach is typically used for DHC. A reverse question mark incision in made on the affected side (**Fig. 1**) and muscle and tissue are then dissected down to the cranium (**Fig. 2**). Burr holes are made and connected to create a bone flap of at least 15 cm to prevent brain herniation and shear forces at the bone edges (**Fig. 3**). The dura is then incised in a stellate fashion leaving the brain exposed (**Fig. 4**).[28] In patients

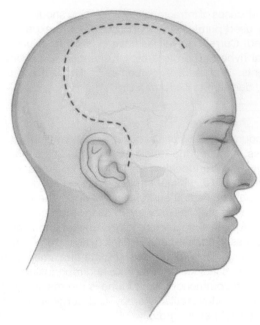

Fig. 1. Skin incision. After the head is shaved and prepared, a large reverse question mark incision is made, beginning at the zygoma extending far behind the ear, then curving a few centimeters lateral to the sagittal suture, anteriorly to the hairline. (*From* Jandial R. Trauma Flap: Decompressive Hemicraniectomy. In: Core Techniques in Operative Neurosurgery (Second Edition). Elsevier; 2019:59-62.)

surviving the acute phase, the defect from the DHC is repaired with a cranioplasty at a later date.

Expert postoperative care following a DHC is critical in ensuring optimal patient outcomes. Patients are admitted to the intensive care unit following the procedure and routine management for prevention of cerebral edema should be initated.[29] Specific care indicated following a DHC includes initiation of flap precautions. Flap precautions include signage and correct patient positioning to avoid pressure on the flap. Postoperative complications are significant requiring acute monitoring for seizures, infection, and cerebral spinal fluid (CSF) leakage.[29–31]

COMPLICATIONS

Complications associated with DHC are widely reported in the literature. In the patient who has had a DHC due to MCE, seizures, hydrocephalus, and hemorrhagic progression of the infarct occur most frequently.[27,31,32] Postoperative seizures are a significant complication with up to half of the patients experiencing seizures in the postoperative period. Management of seizures is dictated by current guidelines.[33]

Hydrocephalus is another common complication occurring in 25.5% of patients undergoing DHC for ischemic stroke. Early cranioplasty may reduce the risk of hydrocephalus, although the timing of cranioplasty is controversial with differing recommendations on the benefits of late versus early cranioplasty.[11,27,32]

Similar to other neurosurgical procedures, DHC in the presence of coagulopathy is associated with an increased risk of complications. Hemorrhagic progression of MCA

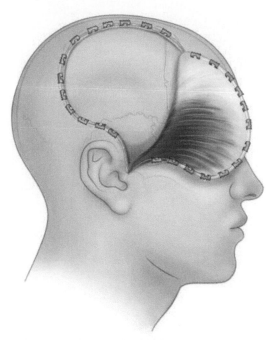

Fig. 2. Muscle and soft tissue dissection. The incision is carried through the subcutaneous tissue, including the temporalis, down to the cranium. The musculocutaneous flap is reflected anteriorly and fixed with scalp hooks. (*From* Jandial R. Trauma Flap: Decompressive Hemicraniectomy. In: Core Techniques in Operative Neurosurgery (Second Edition). Elsevier; 2019:59-62.)

infarcts occurs in approximately a quarter of the cases. Pathophysiological changes as a result of increased intracranial pressure (ICP) and coagulopathy are suspected as causative factors.[31]

A less frequent complication of DHC is syndrome of the trephined. The sinking of the scalp due to the removal of bone leads to fall of the scalp and subsequent clinical manifestations. The prevalence of this syndrome varies across the literature with reports of occurrence between 1% and 40%.[27,30,31] The syndrome is associated with a variety of complaints including motor weakness, headaches, dizziness, pain, and cognitive decline. Cranioplasty repairs the defect, although recommendations for timing of cranioplasty to the reduce complications of DHC are inconclusive in the literature.[34] In a meta-analysis evaluating timing of cranioplasty with neurological symptoms, early cranioplasty was associated with improved neurologic function.[32] Other studies have not supported this finding.[34]

Traumatic injury to the unprotected cranium following DHC is an unfortunate but preventable complication. The removal of a large portion of the skull leaves the brain unprotected. Care to prevent injury is critical and includes flap precautions while in the hospital. Until definitive correction of the bone defect is achieved via cranioplasty, patient use of a protective helmet on discharge is recommended.[27,29]

CONTROVERSY

Accurate assessment to determine which patients will benefit from DHC is necessary to provide comprehensive stroke care. Controversy associated with DHC is

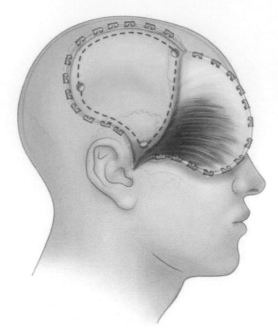

Fig. 3. Burr holes and bone flap. Several burr holes (at least three) are made to create a bone flap that is at least 10 cm × 15 cm. Bone flaps smaller than this would not sufficiently decompress the brain and reduce ICP. (*From* Jandial R. Trauma Flap: Decompressive Hemicraniectomy. In: Core Techniques in Operative Neurosurgery (Second Edition). Elsevier; 2019:59-62.)

extensively documented in the literature.[35–41] The chief concern and resultant controversy is linked to quality of life assessments post-procedure. Other areas of controversy include timing of the procedure, patient selection, and alternative therapies.

Quality of life, and not only survival, has emerged as an important concept when the decision to perform a DHC is considered.[35–40] The determination of what constitutes a favorable outcome is subjective and controversial. An evaluation of neurologic disability is measured using the mRS[42] (**Table 1**).The mRS is a 7-point scale ranging from 0 (no symptoms) to 6 (death). An mRS score of ≤3, indicating patient independence, is generally accepted to represent a favorable outcome, whereas an mRS ≥4 results in patient dependence requiring assistance for daily activities and represents an unfavorable outcome.

The classification of the dichotomy differs in the literature leading to controversy surrounding the assessment of quality of life following DHC. Studies examining DHC in stroke patients defining a favorable outcome as an mRS score of ≤3 found no statistical difference between favorable and unfavorable outcomes in patients who underwent a DHC.[6–8] The DESTINY II trial[43] defined a favorable outcome as an mRS of ≤4 and reported a decrease in unfavorable outcomes in the DHC group compared with the medical management only group. The distinction is relevant in treatment decisions as the practical experience of disability is based on individual values and beliefs. This is apparent when examining the differing perceptions of provider and patient. Asking patients retrospectively if they would have agreed to a procedure, even knowing the outcome was not optimal is known as retrospective consent.[44] Studies assessing retrospective consent are of interest in the DHC

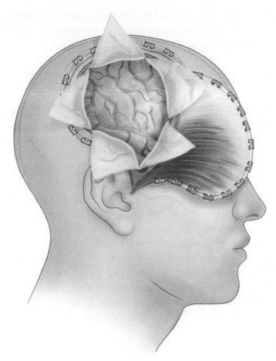

Fig. 4. Durotomy. The dura is opened slowly with multiple radial incisions (in a stellate fashion) to provide maximal cerebral decompression. (*From* Jandial R. Trauma Flap: Decompressive Hemicraniectomy. In: Core Techniques in Operative Neurosurgery (Second Edition). Elsevier; 2019:59-62.)

literature. Patients, particularly older patients, viewed an mRS $\leq$4 as an acceptable outcome, even though they were not fully independent in many cases.[19,37,39] This finding contradicts the perceptions of physicians who viewed an mRS $\geq$4 as an unfavorable outcomes.[37,38] An individual assessment of patient disability acceptance and

Table 1	
Modified Rankin scale	
Score	**Description**
0	No symptoms
1	No significant disability despite symptoms; able to perform all usual duties and activities
2	Slight disability; unable to perform all previous activities but able to look after own affairs without assistance
3	Moderate disability; requiring some help but able to walk without assistance
4	Moderately severe disability; unable to walk with assistance and unable to attend to own bodily needs without assistance
5	Severe disability; bedridden, incontinent, and requires constant nursing care and attention
6	Death

Data from: Robertson FC, Dasenbrock HH, Gormley W. Decompressive Hemicraniectomy for Stroke in Older Adults: A Review. *Journal of Neurology and Neuromedicine*. 2017;2(1):1-7. https://doi.org/10.29245/2572.942x/2017/2.942x/2017/1.1103.

defined goals of care is important topics for family discussions before proceeding with a DHC. Presentation of all options available, and predicted outcomes, is important considerations in the decision-making process.

CURRENT EVIDENCE

With publications demonstrating a decrease in mortality after DHC, utilization of DHC in stroke patients increased.[42] The significant morbidity and disability as a result of DHC prompted a closer investigation of its use for all stroke patients. Alternative treatment options that decreased mortality without significant disability were investigated, most notably the use of endovascular mechanical thrombectomy (MT). Previous studies have demonstrated that early revascularization of the penumbra with endovascular MT decreases mortality without an increase in severe disability.[45–47] The development of MCE was reduced after MT, which consequentially decreased the need for DHC.[4,25,47,48] Results of the THRACE trial demonstrated improved patient function when endovascular MT combined with standard intravenous thrombolysis was used in the treatment of stroke compared with thrombolysis alone. No increase in mortality was observed between the two groups.[48] The increased availability of endovascular MT has correlated with a decrease in DHC in the treatment of strokes. Current guidelines for ischemic stroke recommend thrombolysis followed by endovascular MT with a stent retriever to reduce the risk of MCE if specific criteria, including functional status, CT characteristics, and resource accessibility, are met.[21]

PATIENT PREDICTORS

Evidence-based guidelines exist for utilization of DHC but reveal the need for further research as advanced technologies continue to enhance outcomes in the ischemic stroke patient.[21] Not all stroke patients will develop MCE requiring DHC. Even when indicated, DHC may not be the best option for individual patients. A careful decision-making process to determine which patients are at risk of developing MCE and which should undergo DHC is recommended.[23,36,41] Assessment for patient predictors is recommended to guide the decision-making process.

Many factors contribute to the decision to perform DHC, including CT characteristics, timing of the procedure, and patient expectations. All are important considerations when intervention with a DHC is contemplated. Patients with predictors signifying high risk for development of MCE may benefit from early DHC. Patients who, despite standard therapy and MT, experience progressive neurologic deterioration may also benefit from DHC.[21]

Clinical predictors identifying individuals most at risk for development of MCE are found in the extant literature. An important predictor, large stroke volume, is associated with the development of MCE.[24,35,20] Assessment of CT characteristics using validated tools, such as the Alberta Stroke Program Early CT Score (ASPECTS), facilitates decision-making by assessing individual criteria rather than relying on a generalized treatment approach for all ischemic strokes (**Fig. 5**). The ASPECTS tool assesses ischemic changes present on head CT and predicts patient outcomes. An ASPECTS score is calculated based on the assessment of structures within the MCA vascular territory. Any evidence of early ischemia observed in defined regions results in a subtraction of one point from the 10-point scale.[49] The scale's benefit is in identifying patients in whom an independent recovery despite treatment is unlikely.[49,50] An ASPECTS score of 10 represents a normal CT. More favorable patient outcomes are associated with a higher score. A score of 0 is the result of diffuse ischemic changes throughout the MCA territory. Unfavorable functional outcome at

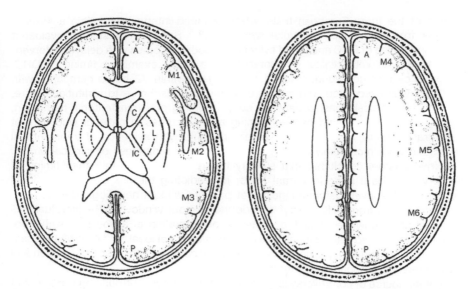

Fig. 5. ASPECTS study form. A, anterior circulation; C, caudate; IC, internal capsule; I, insular ribbon; L, lentiform; M2, MCA cortex lateral to insular ribbon; M3, posterior MCA cortex; MCA, middle cerebral artery; MI, anterior MCA cortex; P, posterior circulation; M4, M5, and M6 are anterior, lateral, and posterior MCA territories immediately superior to MI, M2, and M3, rostral to basal ganglia. Subcortical structures are allotted 3 points (C, L, and 1C). MCA cortex is allotted 7 points (insular cortex, MI, M2, M3, M4, M5, and M6). (*Reprinted with permission from* Elsevier, The Lancet, 2000, 355 (9216), 1670-1674.)

3 months as well as symptomatic hemorrhage is predicted with a score less than or equal to seven.[50]

Advanced age has been reported to negatively impact patient outcomes.[41,44,50] Studies demonstrating a survival benefit with DHC in younger patients failed to evaluate the effect of age on morbidity and mortality.[6–8] These studies found that in patients ≤60 years of age, DHC reduced the risk of death and the risk of severe disability (mRS ≥ 4). Patients older than 60 years of age were excluded from the studies though which left the question of advanced age and outcomes unanswered. Outcomes in patients greater than 60 years of age following a DHC are found in the literature.[42,50] The DESTINY II trial demonstrated a reduction in overall mortality and a decrease in severe disability (mRS ≥ 4) at 6 months post-procedure compared with medical management in patients greater than 60 years of age. After 12 months though, only 6% of patients greater than 60 years of age had an mRS score of ≤ 3. This is compared with the original DESTINY trial which found 47% of younger patients had an mRS of less than 3 at 12 months post-procedure. A significant reduction of disability (mRS < 3) was not demonstrated in either study.[6] In another study, 1 year survival in older patients was 55% with 29% of survivors requiring institutional long-term care.[44] The clear mortality benefit in all age patients but an associated higher incidence of unfavorable outcomes in patients greater than 60 years of age warrants consideration of age in the decision-making process.[40,42]

The timing of DHC and the presence of progressive neurological symptoms also features prominently in the decision-making process. Current guidelines recommend consideration of DHC performed within 48 hours of the onset of stroke symptoms in patients with neurological deterioration.[21] The time window is based on the enrollment criteria of the three European trials, which required intervention within a 48-hour window from the onset of stroke symptoms.[6–8] Subsequent studies evaluated extending timing of DHC and found evidence of poor outcomes with delayed intervention in patients with clinical deterioration. In a study examining timing of DHC, Dasenbrock and colleagues[20] found that surgery within 72 hours compared with 48 hours was associated with a poor outcome and discharge to institutional care. Of note was the relationship between surgical timing and transtentorial herniation. No association was found between timing and outcomes in patients who did not have transtentorial herniation. Conversely, patients with evidence of transtentorial herniation were more likely to have a poor outcome regardless of surgical timing. The investigators concluded that surgery before herniation, rather than timing of surgery, may be a more important factor in predicting the risk of poor functional outcomes. The investigators suggest that patients without neurologic deterioration may still benefit from DHC even if outside the 48-hour window.[20] The literature has demonstrated, however, that the evidence of herniation is associated with poor patient outcomes so waiting for clinical deterioration is not ideal.[21,20] A careful assessment of patient and family acceptance of disability coupled with close observation and rapid intervention should guide therapy.

Another source of controversy is found in societal factors surrounding treatment of stroke. The evidence of socioeconomic disparities in stroke survival is found in the literature.[15,51,52] Access to advanced stroke care is associated with better outcomes but is not accessible to all communities. A recent systematic review found that patients admitted directly to a comprehensive stroke center had significantly better outcomes compared with patients who were directed to a primary stroke center followed by transfer.[15,21,51] Admission to a teaching hospital is associated with earlier DHC.[41,20] The inaccessibility of advanced care found in specialized facilities results in a delay in treatment and, as previously noted, delayed DHC is associated with unfavorable patient outcomes. The delay in definitive care places patients without access to state-of-the-art facilities at a disadvantage. Improving patient access and health disparities have the potential to dramatically affect patient survival and functional status.[21]

CASE STUDY

A 50-year-old man with left-sided hemiparesis that began 90 minutes ago presented to the emergency department of a large, teaching hospital. The hospital was certified as comprehensive stroke center and a stroke code was initiated. The patient's National Institutes of Health Stroke Scale score on admission was 10. A non-contrast head CT revealed findings consistent with a right MCA stroke. Assessment of the

---

Box 1
Key factors for favorable patient outcomes following decompressive hemicraniectomy

Age <60

ASPECTS score >7

Admission to a teaching hospital

Admission to a comprehensive stroke center

Patient-centered discussions

Box 2
Postoperative decompressive hemicraniectomy care

- Close assessment for neurological deterioration
- Correction of hypotension or hypovolemia to maintain systemic perfusion levels needed to support organ function.
- Supplementation of oxygen to maintain oxygen saturation >94%.
- Avoidance of hypo/hyperglycemia
- Intracranial monitoring is recommended to guide therapy and is helpful in determination of the need for secondary DHC.
- Osmotic therapy is indicated for patients with clinical deterioration from cerebral edema.
- Hypothermia or barbiturates are not recommended for ischemic swelling.
- Flap assessment/flap precautions
- Seizure precautions
- Deep vein thrombosis prophylaxis
- Wound care and monitoring for infection

Data from Powers W, Rabinstein A, Ackerson T, et al. Guidelines for the Early Management of Patients With Acute Ischemic Stroke: 2019 Update to the 2018 Guidelines for the Early Management of Acute Ischemic Stroke: A Guideline for Healthcare Professionals From the American Heart Association/American Stroke Association. *Stroke.* 2019;50(12). https://www.ahajournals.org/doi/full/10.1161/STR.0000000000000211.

---

imaging estimated an ASPECTS score of 8. The patient was treated with IV thrombolysis within 3 hours of the last known well time without incident. After neurosurgical evaluation, it was determined the patient would benefit from endovascular MT. The patient was admitted to the neuroscience intensive care unit from the interventional suite post-procedure and an intracranial pressure device was placed. Medical management of ICP was initiated but despite maximal efforts, neurological deterioration progressed with sustained ICP $\geq$ 18. A repeat head CT 24 hours after admission demonstrated progressive edema but no signs of transtentorial herniation. A family meeting was scheduled to discuss treatment options. Understanding the risks of severe disability or death, the patient's wife agreed to proceed with a DHC. A right DHC was performed resulting in the relief of intracranial hypertension and improvement in the patient's neurological status. The patient continued to improve and was discharged with an mRS of 4 to a stroke rehabilitation facility 10 days after admission. Follow-up at 6 and 12 months demonstrated an improved functional status with an mRS of 3. Both the patient and wife reported satisfaction with their decision to proceed with DHC and are content with the patient's current functional status. This patient represents the ideal patient for DHC **Box 1** and supports advanced, comprehensive stroke management in efforts to improve patient outcomes **Box 2**.

SUMMARY

Treatment of the stroke patient is complex and requires thoughtful consideration of known risks and benefits. Both medical and surgical interventions are used in the management of ischemic stroke. Identified clinical predictors that impact patient outcomes should be carefully evaluated before consideration of any intervention.

The literature has extensively demonstrated that DHC decreases patient mortality but frequently results in severe disability, particularly in patients greater than 60 years of age.[6–10,41,50] Acceptance of disability differs significantly among providers, patients, and families. Thus, treatment decisions should be patient-centered and considered within the context of what the patient and family deem an acceptable outcome.

Advances in neurosurgical interventions and postoperative care have dramatically changed the management of ischemic stroke but socioeconomic factors limit access to all stroke patients resulting in a disparity of care. DHC is a life-saving procedure and is a reasonable option in select patients with ischemic stroke. Access to advanced, comprehensive care must be a priority goal in the management of stroke.

CLINICS CARE POINTS

- DHC decreases mortality by relieving increased ICP and improving perfusion.
- Quality of life, particularly in the elderly population, may be compromised following DHC.
- Optimal timing of DHC continues to be debated in the literature.
- Assessment for patient predictors is recommended to guide the decision-making process.
- Adherence to published guidelines for management of the stroke patient can improve patient outcomes.

DISCLOSURE

The author has nothing to disclose.

REFERENCES

1. Feigin VL, Brainin M, Norrving B, et al. World stroke organization (WSO): global stroke fact sheet 2022. Int J Stroke 2022;17(1):18–29.
2. Ekker MS, Boot EM, Singhal AB, et al. Epidemiology, aetiology, and management of ischaemic stroke in young adults. Lancet Neurol 2018;17(9):790–801.
3. Picetti E, Caspani ML, Iaccarino C, et al. Intracranial pressure monitoring after primary decompressive craniectomy in traumatic brain injury: a clinical study. Acta Neurochirurgica 2017;159(4):615–22.
4. Sandroni C, Cronberg T, Sekhon M. Brain injury after cardiac arrest: pathophysiology, treatment, and prognosis. Intensive Care Med 2021;47(12):1393–414.
5. Vedantam A, Robertson CS, Gopinath SP, et al. Quantitative cerebral blood flow using xenon-enhanced CT after decompressive craniectomy in traumatic brain injury. J Neurosurg 2018;129(1):241–6.
6. Juttler E, Schwab S, Schmiedek P, et al. Decompressive surgery for the treatment of malignant infarction of the middle cerebral artery (DESTINY). Stroke 2007; 38(9):2518–25.
7. Vahedi K, Vicaut E, Mateo J, et al. Sequential-design, multicenter, randomized, controlled trial of early decompressive craniectomy in malignant middle cerebral artery infarction (DECIMAL trial). Stroke 2007;38(9):2506–17.
8. Hofmeijer J, Kappelle LJ, Algra A, et al. Surgical decompression for space-occupying cerebral infarction (the Hemicraniectomy after Middle Cerebral Artery infarction with Life-threatening Edema Trial [HAMLET]): a multicentre, open, randomised trial. Lancet Neurol 2009;8(4):326–33.

9. Vahedi K, Hofmeijer J, Juettler E, et al. Early decompressive surgery in malignant infarction of the middle cerebral artery: a pooled analysis of three randomised controlled trials. Lancet Neurol 2007;6(3):215–22.
10. Back L, Nagaraja V, Kapur A, et al. Role of decompressive hemicraniectomy in extensive middle cerebral artery strokes: a meta-analysis of randomised trials. Intern Med J 2015;45(7):711–7.
11. Beez T, Steiger HJ. Impact of randomized controlled trials on neurosurgical practice in decompressive craniectomy for ischemic stroke. Neurosurg Rev 2018; 42(1):133–7.
12. Gross CG. A hole in the head : more tales in the history of neuroscience. Cambridge, MA: Mit Press; 2012.
13. Kushner DS, Verano JW, Titelbaum AR. Trepanation procedures/outcomes: comparison of prehistoric Peru with other ancient, medieval, and American civil war cranial surgery. World Neurosurg 2018;114:245–51.
14. Kolias AG, Viaroli E, Rubiano AM, et al. The current status of decompressive craniectomy in traumatic brain injury. Curr Trauma Rep 2018;4(4):326–32.
15. Khan Zubair Mustafa, Safdar Zehra, Syed Ahmad F, et al. Outcome & complications of decompressive craniectomy with expansion duroplasty in severe head injury. Pakistan J Neurol Surg 2022;26(2):194–202.
16. Cooper DJ, Rosenfeld JV, Murray L, et al. Decompressive craniectomy in diffuse traumatic brain injury. 2011. Available at: https://www.nejm.org/doi/full/10.1056/NEJMoa1102077. Accessed August 15, 2022.
17. Hutchinson P, Timofeev I, Grainger S, et al. The RESCUEicp decompressive craniectomy trial. Crit Care 2009;13(Suppl 1):P85.
18. Cruz-Flores S, Berge E, Whittle IR. Surgical decompression for cerebral oedema in acute ischaemic stroke. Cochrane Database Syst Rev 2012;1. https://doi.org/10.1002/14651858.cd003435.pub2.
19. Garcia-Estrada E, Morales-Gómez JA, Romero-González M, et al. Decompressive craniectomy for hemispheric infarction in a low-income population. World Neurosurg 2021;156:e152–9.
20. Dasenbrock HH, Robertson FC, Vaitkevicius H, et al. Timing of decompressive hemicraniectomy for stroke. Stroke 2017;48(3):704–11.
21. Powers W, Rabinstein A, Ackerson T, et al. Guidelines for the early management of patients with acute ischemic stroke: 2019 update to the 2018 guidelines for the early management of acute ischemic stroke: a guideline for healthcare Professionals from the American Heart association/American stroke association. Stroke 2019;50(12). Available at: https://www.ahajournals.org/doi/full/10.1161/STR.0000000000000211.
22. Rossini Z, Nicolosi F, Angelos GK, et al. The history of decompressive craniectomy in traumatic brain injury. Front Neurol 2019;10. https://doi.org/10.3389/fneur.2019.00458.
23. Lin J, Frontera JA. Decompressive hemicraniectomy for large hemispheric strokes. Stroke 2021;52(4):1500–10.
24. Miao J, Song X, Sun W, et al. Predictors of malignant cerebral edema in cerebral artery infarction: a meta-analysis. J Neurol Sci 2020;409:116607.
25. Rumalla K, Ottenhausen M, Kan P, et al. Recent nationwide impact of mechanical thrombectomy on decompressive hemicraniectomy for acute ischemic stroke. Stroke 2019;50(8):2133–9.
26. Smith M. Refractory intracranial hypertension. Anesth Analgesia 2017;125(6):1999–2008.

27. Sveikata L, Vasung L, El Rahal A, et al. Syndrome of the trephined: clinical spectrum, risk factors, and impact of cranioplasty on neurologic recovery in a prospective cohort. Neurosurg Rev 2021;45(2):1431–43.

28. Jandial R. Trauma flap: decompressive hemicraniectomy. In: Core techniques in operative Neurosurgery. Second Edition. Elsevier; 2019. p. 59–62. Available at: https://www.sciencedirect.com/science/article/pii/B97803235238130001.   Accessed August 2, 2022.

29. Guanci MM. Management of the patient with malignant hemispheric stroke. Crit Care Nurs Clin North America 2020;32(1):51–66.

30. Gopalakrishnan MS, Shanbhag NC, Shukla DP, et al. Complications of decompressive craniectomy. Front Neurol 2018;9. https://doi.org/10.3389/fneur.2018.00977.

31. Mraček J, Mork J, Dostal J, et al. Complications following decompressive craniectomy. J Neurol Surg A Cent Eur Neurosurg 2021;82(5):437–45.

32. Malcolm JG, Rindler RS, Chu JK, et al. Early cranioplasty is associated with greater neurological improvement: a systematic review and meta-analysis. Neurosurgery 2018;82(3):278–88.

33. American Academy of Neurology. Evidence-based guideline: management of an unprovoked first seizure in adults 2015. Available at: https://www.aan.com/Guidelines/home/GuidelineDetail/687 www.aan.com.

34. Aloraidi A, Alkhaibary A, Alharbi A, et al. Effect of cranioplasty timing on the functional neurological outcome and postoperative complications. Surg Neurol Int 2021;12:264.

35. Honeybul S, Ho KM, Gillett G. Outcome following decompressive hemicraniectomy for malignant cerebral infarction. Stroke 2015;46(9):2695–8.

36. Mahanes D. Ethical concerns caring for the stroke patient. Crit Care Nurs Clin North America 2020;32(1):121–33.

37. Budhdeo S, Kolias AG, Clark DJ, et al. A retrospective cohort study to assess patient and physician reported outcome measures after decompressive hemicraniectomy for malignant middle cerebral artery. Stroke Cureus 2017. https://doi.org/10.7759/cureus.1237.

38. Neugebauer H, Creutzfeldt CJ, Hemphill JC, et al. Attitudes of physicians toward disability and treatment in malignant MCA infarction. Neurocrit Care 2014;21(1):27–34.

39. Ragoschke-Schumm A, Junk C, Lesmeister M, et al. Retrospective consent to hemicraniectomy after malignant stroke among the elderly, despite impaired functional outcome. Cerebrovasc Dis 2015;40(5–6):286–92.

40. Lu X, Huang B, Zheng J, et al. Decompressive craniectomy for the treatment of malignant infarction of the middle cerebral artery. Scientific Rep 2014;4(1).

41. Moody K, Santos D, Stein LK, et al. Decompressive hemicraniectomy for acute ischemic stroke in the US: characteristics and outcomes. J Stroke Cerebrovasc Dis 2021;30(5):105703.

42. Robertson FC, Dasenbrock HH, Gormley W. Decompressive hemicraniectomy for stroke in older adults: a review. J Neurol Neuromedicine 2017;2(1):1–7.

43. Jüttler E, Unterberg A, Woitzik J, et al. Hemicraniectomy in older patients with extensive middle-cerebral-artery stroke. New Engl J Med 2014;370(12):1091–100.

44. Fehnel CR, Lee Y, Wendell LC, et al. Utilization of long-term care after decompressive hemicraniectomy for severe stroke among older patients. Aging Clin Exp Res 2016;29(4):631–8.

45. Albers GW, Marks MP, Kemp S, et al. Thrombectomy for stroke at 6 to 16 hours with selection by perfusion imaging. New Engl J Med 2018;378(8):708–18.
46. Nogueira RG, Jadhav AP, Haussen DC, et al. Thrombectomy 6 to 24 hours after stroke with a mismatch between deficit and infarct. New Engl J Med 2018;378(1): 11–21.
47. Berkhemer O, Fransen P, Beumer D, et al. A randomized trial of intraarterial treatment for acute ischemic stroke. New Engl J Med 2015;372(4):394.
48. Bracard S, Ducrocq X, Mas JL, et al. Mechanical thrombectomy after intravenous alteplase versus alteplase alone after stroke (THRACE): a randomised controlled trial. Lancet Neurol 2016;15(11):1138–47.
49. Barber PA, Demchuk AM, Zhang J, et al. Validity and reliability of a quantitative computed tomography score in predicting outcome of hyperacute stroke before thrombolytic therapy. The Lancet 2000;355(9216):1670–4.
50. Sair H. Alberta stroke programme early CT score (ASPECTS) | Radiology Reference Article | Radiopaedia.org. Radiopaedia. 2022. https://radiopaedia.org/ articles/alberta-stroke-programme-early-ct-score-aspects?lang=us. Accessed August 13, 2022.
51. Ismail M, Armoiry X, Tau N, et al. Mothership versus drip and ship for thrombectomy in patients who had an acute stroke: a systematic review and meta-analysis. J NeuroInterventional Surg 2018;11(1):14–9.
52. Vivanco-Hidalgo RM, Ribera A, Abilleira S. Association of socioeconomic status with ischemic stroke survival. Stroke 2019. https://doi.org/10.1161/strokeaha. 119.026607.

Invasive Neuromonitoring in the Stroke Patient

Carey Heck, PhD, CRNP, AGACNP-BC, CNRN

KEYWORDS

- Neurosurgery • Multimodal monitoring • Stroke • Intracranial pressure
- Brain oxygenation • Microdialysis

KEY POINTS

- Monitoring devices such as intraparenchymal monitors and external ventricular devices are routinely used to detect and intervene in instances of increased intracranial pressure (ICP) in the stroke patient.
- ICP monitoring alone does not identify ischemic changes that herald patient deterioration.
- Changes in the brain cerebral oxygenation and metabolism indicating hypoxia and ischemia occur despite the presence of normal ICP and CPP values.
- Multimodality monitoring augments data derived from ICP and is advantageous in preventing poor patient outcomes.

INTRODUCTION

With advances in technology, the options to manage patients with neurologic injuries are often complex. Critical care management of neurologic injury has historically focused on the prevention of secondary ischemic injury through aggressive management of intracranial pressure (ICP) and maintenance of adequate cerebral perfusion pressure (CPP).[1-4] The concept of ICP was first introduced in 1783 by Scottish physician, Dr. Monro, who described the skull as a rigid box with a fixed volume that was composed of blood, brain tissue, and cerebral spinal fluid (CSF). In 1824, Scottish surgeon, Dr. Kellie, further expanded on this hypothesis by noting that an increase in the volume of one component resulted in a decrease in the volume of the other components. The work by these early physicians is now well known as the Monro–Kellie hypothesis and has significant implications when discussing and managing ICP and invasive neuromonitoring.[4]

Invasive neuromonitoring has been the mainstay of neurocritical care management for centuries, particularly in the management of patients with traumatic brain injury and subarachnoid hemorrhage (SAH).[1-6] Much of the literature supporting invasive neuromonitoring is found in the traumatic brain injury (TBI) population. Although not as

Adult-Gerontology Acute Care Nurse Practitioner Program, Thomas Jefferson University, 901 Walnut Street, Suite 815, Philadelphia, PA 19107, USA
E-mail address: Carey.Heck@Jefferson.edu

Crit Care Nurs Clin N Am 35 (2023) 83–94
https://doi.org/10.1016/j.cnc.2022.10.006
0899-5885/23/© 2022 Elsevier Inc. All rights reserved.

pronounced as in TBI literature, the use of invasive neuromonitoring in stroke patient is significant.[7–10]

Annually, approximately 795,000 individuals in the United States experience a new or recurrent stroke. The vast majority (87%) of these strokes are ischemic.[6,11] The annual incidence of hemorrhagic stroke due to SAH is estimated at 9.1 days per 100,000. Up to 30% of these have poor outcomes, most frequently as a result of vasospasm and delayed cerebral ischemia.[6–8] Even with standard management, a percentage of stroke patients will develop life-threatening complications requiring complex treatments to reduce mortality and preserve functional status. Early identification of ischemic changes allows for early intervention and is key to reducing poor outcomes. Identifying changes not only in ICP but early ischemic changes as well support comprehensive care of stroke patients. The literature demonstrates increasing utilization of technology capable of assessing brain oxygen levels and brain metabolism.[8–11] Monitoring these important dynamics has the potential to improve patient outcomes. Understanding the advantages, disadvantages, and indications for use of invasive neuromonitoring in the stroke patient facilitates optimal patient care.

Despite the unwavering reliance on ICP monitoring, it is essential to observe that significant controversy exists in the literature surrounding this technology.[2,5,6,12,13] Controversy exists concerning the timing and placement of devices.[6,7,14,15] The literature notes controversy surrounding the use of single-device ICP monitoring versus multimodality monitoring.[3,14–18] Finally, as a result of the Benchmark Evidence from South American Trials: Treatment of Intracranial Pressure (BEST TRIP) trial,[19] substantial debate has been generated concerning the ultimate benefit of ICP monitoring in specific patient populations.[8,9,11,16–18]

RATIONALE FOR INVASIVE NEUROMONITORING

The care of the stroke patient is multidimensional. The overarching goal of neurocritical care management is to prevent secondary brain ischemia.[1,6,12,15] This is particularly true in stroke when salvage of the penumbra with the restoration of brain perfusion is the primary aim.[4,5] The assessment of ICP and CPP is the most prevalent intervention in invasive neuromonitoring and is standard practice in neurocritical care management. Increased ICP has repeatedly been demonstrated to compromise cerebral blood flow leading to cerebral hypoxia, ischemia, and death.[4,12,17,20] The negative consequences of increased ICP include increased mortality and morbidity.[1,12,17] Conversely, aggressive management and control of ICP has been demonstrated to result in improved neurologic outcomes in patients with TBI and subarachnoid hemorrhage.[1,4,9,21]

The goals of management are generally accepted as maintenance of ICP less than 20 mm Hg with a CPP goal of 60 to 70 mm Hg.[1,4,16,22–24] Ultimately, the ICP and CPP reference ranges should be individualized for each patient, taking into consideration underlying abnormality and goals of treatment.[4,16,18,22,23] In a patient with a stroke, aggressive management and control of ICP are warranted. However, ICP monitoring alone does not identify ischemic changes that herald patient deterioration. Additional devices that monitor brain oxygen and metabolic changes allow for timely interventions before clinical or ICP changes are noted.

Monitoring of intracranial pressure[1,14,20,22,23]

- Allows for the rapid recognition of elevated ICP
- Ensures maintenance of optimal CPP
- Assesses the efficacy of therapeutic measures
- Evaluates the evolution of brain injury

INDICATIONS FOR INVASIVE NEUROMONITORING

A variety of disease processes and neurologic conditions warrant the use of invasive neuromonitoring.[2,4,14–19,21–23] Patients with severe TBI and patients with SAH as a result of cerebral aneurysmal rupture are routinely managed with invasive neuromonitoring. For the patient with ischemic stroke, reperfusion therapies coupled with specialized stroke unit care is routine. It is only when there is concern for malignant edema or the patient presents in extremis that a role for invasive monitoring is found in the ischemic stroke patient.[5] Subsequently, TBI and SAH dominate research and case study literature.[1,7,11,13]

Much of the extant literature on ICP monitoring is focused on the patient with severe TBI. The propensity of literature on this specific population, along with the adoption of international guidelines and standardized protocols, has resulted in the acceptance of ICP monitoring as the mainstay for the care of patients with severe TBI at most large trauma centers in developed countries.[1,2,18,24] The use of external ventricular devices (EVDs) for temporary or permanent CSF diversion is recommended in symptomatic patients with chronic hydrocephalus following SAH.[6,20] Recommendations for ICP monitoring are also noted in evidence-based guidelines for intracerebral hemorrhage.[11,25]

The most common indications include use in patients with[1,2,8,14,22,23]

- TBI
- SAH
- Intracerebral hemorrhage
- Obstructive hydrocephalus

Other indications include patients with

- Cerebral infections
- Congenital abnormalities
- Mass lesions
- Hepatic failure

INTRACRANIAL MONITORING OPTIONS

In patients who are at risk for increased ICP, the ICP and CPP monitoring are recommended as part of protocol-driven care.[10,19] A variety of devices are available to monitor ICP. Device selection is dictated by the patient's presentation and desired device function, practitioner preference, and institutional policies and is ideally driven by the current best evidence.[10,13,14,20]

ICP monitors are classified based on their ultimate location within the brain (**Fig. 1**) and their function (monitoring of ICP alone or monitoring and therapy). Devices inserted directly into the parenchyma are commonly referred to as intraparenchymal monitors (IPM) in the literature. A catheter inserted into the cerebral ventricle and attached to a transducer system allows for monitoring of ICP as well as continuous or intermittent drainage of CSF.[1,3–6] The latter devices are collectively referred to as EVDs in the literature. IPMs and EVDs are used most frequently in the clinical setting[14,20]

The most serious complications for stroke patients are evolving ischemic changes due to malignant cerebral edema or vasospasm. In the stroke patient, delayed cerebral ischemia (DCI) is a serious complication resulting in significant death and disability.[16] In the subarachnoid hemorrhage patient, DCI typically occurs 4 to 21 days after aneurysmal rupture.[6,7,13] The patient with an ischemic stroke similarly

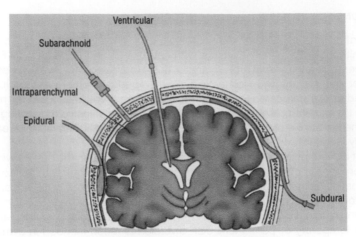

Fig. 1. Placement of invasive neuromonitoring devices. (*Adapted from* Kerr M, Crago EA. Nursing management: acute intracranial problems. In: Lewis SM, Heitkemper MM, Dirksen SR, editors. Medical-surgical nursing: assessment and management of clinical problems, 6th edition. St Louis (MO): CV Mosby; 2004. p. 1918; with permission.)

is at risk for malignant edema which also, if detected early, can be aggressively managed. The occurrence of DCI is unpredictable so efforts to identify ischemic changes early are beneficial.[7] Invasive neuromonitoring permits trending of ICP and monitoring of cerebral oxygenation and metabolism. Brain tissue oxygen monitoring in the management of neuroscience patients has been a topic of interest in the neuro-critical care literature for decades.[8,17,26] Advocates of continuous brain oxygen monitoring argue that changes in brain cerebral oxygenation indicating hypoxia and ischemia occur despite the presence of normal ICP and CPP values.[3,8,15] Cerebral oxygenation and metabolism monitoring represent advanced technology that has the potential to improve patient outcomes when coupled with ICP monitoring.

ADVANTAGES AND DISADVANTAGES OF INVASIVE NEUROMONITORING

The decision to use technology is based on consideration of many factors. Patient presentation and the goals of therapy will quite frequently drive the decision for device choice. The technical expertise of the practitioner as well as institutional culture and policies will also be significant considerations. The advantages and disadvantages of the numerous devices available to the practitioner must also be deliberated because these often overlap with the previously mentioned considerations. **Table 1** summarizes the advantages, disadvantages, and indications for the most commonly used invasive neuromonitoring devices.

Device Insertion

Measurement of ICP is achieved by the insertion of devices into the brain parenchyma or the cerebral ventricles.[7,20,25,31,32] Choice of the device is based on whether the ultimate goal of management is ICP monitoring alone (for instance in a patient with TBI). In this scenario, placement of an IPM would be appropriate. If, however, the management goal is ICP monitoring and drainage of CSF or blood (for instance, in a patient with SAH or a patient with hydrocephalus), then an EVD would be a more appropriate choice.

Table 1
Advantages, disadvantages, and indications for invasive neuromonitors

Type of Monitor	Location	Advantages	Disadvantages	Indications
Intraparenchymal Monitor (IPM)	Parenchyma	Ease of placement Less infectious complications	Cannot be recalibrated once placed Fiberoptics are easily damaged Cost	Guides therapy for patients requiring ICP monitoring or patients with imminent brain herniation
External Ventricular Device (EVD)	Ventricles	"Gold standard" Most reliable and accurate Monitoring and therapy via drainage of CSF and blood Easily recalibrated in situ	Technically challenging to insert in certain clinical situations Higher risk of complication including infection and hemorrhage Obstruction possibility	Guides therapy for patients requiring ICP monitoring or patients with imminent brain herniation
PbtO2	Parenchyma	Early detection of cerebral ischemia Low rates of complications	Cerebral oxygenation dependent on catheter placement Use with other monitoring recommended	Patients at risk for ischemia or hypoxia
SjvO2	Jugular bulb	Early detection of cerebral ischemia	Catheter tip malposition Higher risk of complication including infection and hemorrhage Frequent recalibrations	Patients at risk for ischemia or hypoxia
Microdialysis	Parenchyma	Early detection of cerebral metabolic changes	Complexity of data Normal values and thresholds for treatment are not defined Use with other monitoring recommended	Patients at risk for cerebral ischemia, hypoxia, and cerebral energy dysfunction

Data from Refs. 6,8,14–16,20,21,27–30

A basic understanding of the anatomic landmarks for device insertion is necessary and is henceforth described. Insertion of an intracranial monitor is performed in the operating room or at the patient's bedside, although institutional variations may be significant and will be dictated by those policies and procedures. Insertion of any invasive neuromonitoring device carries the risk of infection.[4,20,27,31] The procedure is, therefore, conducted adhering to a strict sterile technique. Insertion by a credentialed practitioner may be done using several techniques, although the most common point for ICP monitor insertion is the Kocher point.[32,33]

The Kocher point is located by measuring

- 10.5 to 11 cm back from the nasion (bridge of the nose)
- 2.5 to 3.0 cm lateral to the midline (midpupillary line)

Alternatively, measuring 1 cm anterior of the coronal suture on the midpupillary line is another method to locate the Kocher point.[22,33,34]

External Ventricular Drains

Several types of EVD transducers are available in the clinical setting. These transducers include external strain-gauge, internal strain-gauge, or fiberoptic catheter.[14,18,24,33,34] EVDs can be easily recalibrated, rendering them highly accurate. As noted earlier, EVDs not only allow for the measurement of ICP but also have the added benefit of allowing therapeutic interventions through the drainage of CSF or blood.[12,33,34] For these reasons, EVDs are preferred when hydrocephalus accompanies elevated ICP.[10,34,35]

The literature has noted the advantages of EVDs in the management of both patients with TBI and patients with SAH.[11,25] Hydrocephalus is a common complication in patients with SAH and may occur acutely with the need for urgent treatment. Clinical improvement after placement of an EVD has been demonstrated to improve patient outcomes although controversy exists regarding maintenance and duration of therapy.[27,33–37] The disadvantages of EVDs are evident when one considers the end location of the device. The device is most frequently placed in the lateral ventricle, and placement can be challenging if the ventricle is compressed due to mass effect or collapsed because of a lack of CSF.[13,20] The literature has also noted an increased risk of hemorrhage and infection when compared with IPM.[13,27,31,33–38] Other investigators, however, have noted no difference in the rate of complication between the two device types.[20,35]

Intraparenchymal Monitors

Another method of measuring ICP is through the use of catheters inserted directly into the brain parenchyma. These intraparenchymal monitors (IPM) are used when drainage of CSF is not necessary or when insertion into the ventricle is not possible (in the case of ventricular compression due to cerebral edema, for example). Subdural, subarachnoid, and epidural bolts are used less frequently because of inaccuracies of ICP measurements.[15,26,31] The advantages of IPMs include fewer technical challenges with device placement and theoretically a lower risk of infection. Disadvantages of IPMs include the inability to recalibrate once the device has been placed and the cost compared with EVDs.[14,16,33–35]

Multimodal Monitoring

The concern that ICP monitoring may not confer a benefit has been previously discussed and is the subject of much controversy. Much of the dialogue in the literature argues that ICP monitoring alone should not be the sole source of information on which therapy is guided, but should be incorporated into the arsenal of emerging and promising invasive neuromonitoring devices.[10,18,20,38,39] In addition to ICP monitoring, cerebral oxygenation and metabolism monitoring have been shown in the literature to optimize patient outcomes.[2,7,10,38] The collection and analysis of patient information from multiple sources are referred to as multimodal monitoring.

Multimodal monitoring has been described as a dynamic process that uses a variety of tools to simultaneously monitor multiple cerebral physiologic data.[8,15,18,26,38] The integration of data allows the practitioner to discretely and precisely adjust therapy based on individual changes to a patient's brain physiology.[3,14,18,26] The implementation of multimodal monitoring augments ICP monitoring by detecting early ischemic changes. This is particularly relevant given the goal of stroke management is reperfusion of the penumbra and prevention of further ischemia. In addition, multimodality monitoring has been noted to confer a survival benefit to TBI patients.[2,19,39,40] Although the evidence for multimodal monitoring and improved patient outcomes in the stroke patient is limited, multimodal monitoring seems to offer promise for invasive neuromonitoring options in the care of critically ill neuroscience patients.[3,13,14,16,28,38–40]

Brain Tissue Oxygen Monitoring

Monitoring intracranial volume changes alone, which is the only information derived from IPMs and EVDs, may be inadequate for the practitioner tasked with managing critically ill neuroscience patients. It has been demonstrated that ICP monitoring alone misses the dynamic changes in oxygen delivery and consumption that occur before clinical signs are evident in a patient's assessment.[3,12,17,27,40] Indeed, the use of these devices are not recommended as the sole means of therapy in stroke patients but instead as adjunctive tools along with ICP monitoring.[10]

Additional physiologic information available through monitoring of cerebral oxygenation augments data provided by IPMs and EVDs. Brain tissue oxygenation tension (PbtO2) and jugular venous oxygen consumption (SjvO2) detect cerebral perfusion and hypoxia[16,27,40] PbtO2 is monitored via the insertion of specialized probes inserted adjacent to ICP monitoring catheters. The placement of the $PbtO_2$ catheter may be in the white matter on either the injured or the uninjured side of the brain. Placement on the injured side of the brain provides regional data. Placement on the uninjured side of the brain permits examination of therapy effectiveness and allows for early detection of further ischemic damage.[8,15,26] The ultimate placement is dictated by the cause of neurologic insult and the information desired. The literature defines normal $PbtO_2$ between 25 and 35 mm Hg with the initiation of treatment generally recommended for $PbtO_2$ less than 20 mm Hg.[12,26]

$SjvO_2$ reflects the difference between cerebral oxygen supply and demand and is a useful tool to identify cerebral ischemia. In SjvO2 monitoring, a fiber optic catheter is inserted in the internal jugular vein and provides an assessment of global oxygenation[12,20,29] It too is recommended as part of a multimodal approach to management.[10,12,20] Normal SjvO2 is 55% to 75%. SjvO2 values < 55% suggest cerebral hypoxia or increased metabolic oxygen consumption (CMRO2). SjvO2 desaturation is associated with poor clinical outcomes. Values > 75% indicate increased oxygen delivery or decreased CMRO2.[12,26,29]

Interventions are directed toward improving oxygenation to prevent further ischemia or neuronal death.[16,27,29] These interventions may include strategies to improve hypotension, hypovolemia, or hypoxia.[7,24] Interventions to decrease cerebral metabolism are also important and include sedation, pain management, maintenance of normothermia, and seizure prophylaxis.[24]

Cerebral Microdialysis

Additional insight into pathophysiological processes is possible when cerebral microdialysis is initiated. Data obtained from ICP monitors and brain oxygenation monitors combined with cerebral microdialysis provide important information to guide therapy and minimize secondary ischemic injury.[10,30] With cerebral microdialysis, a specialized catheter is inserted into the brain parenchyma and rests ipsilateral to the injured brain. Placement of the catheter allows for the sampling of neurochemical markers including glucose, lactate, pyruvate, lactate/pyruvate ratio (LPR), and glutamate. Mortality and unfavorable patient outcomes are observed with low glucose levels and/or elevated LPR.[10,27,30] Decisions regarding interventions to optimize CPP and oxygen delivery are facilitated with data derived from cerebral microdialysis enabling a tailored approach to patient care. As with brain oxygenation monitoring, cerebral microdialysis is recommended as part of a multimodal approach to care in patients who are at risk for ischemia, hypoxia, or energy failure.[7,10,30]

Noninvasive Neuromonitoring

The risk of infection with invasive devices is always a concern in patient management. Noninvasive options for neuromonitoring provide estimations of cerebral blood flow (CBF) without the risks of infection or the trauma of invasive procedures. The most common noninvasive monitor is the transcranial ultrasound (TCU) which provides a global assessment.[5,18] Blood flow velocity is measured noninvasively with TCU by emitting and receiving high-frequency energy. The velocity and direction of CBF are reflected in changes in frequency.[5,14,18,28] Its benefit in detecting cerebral vasospasm and potential ischemia in patients with SAH is well documented, however, operator dependency limits its usefulness.[14,28] Near-infrared spectroscopy (NIRS) is an emerging noninvasive tool to measure cerebral oxygenation. NIRS has shown value in detecting time-critical global perfusion changes. Limited studies demonstrating NIRS effectiveness as a tool for advanced monitoring are found in the literature[12,26,28] More research is needed to recommend the use of NIRS routinely in the care of patients with neurologic injury.

CONTROVERSIES IN INVASIVE NEUROMONITORING

As noted earlier, ICP monitoring based on established guidelines is the accepted standard of care in developed countries for the management of patients with TBI, despite a lack of randomized controlled trials.[4,6,14] The findings of the BEST TRIP trial[19] suggested that ICP monitoring was not superior to care based on clinical assessment and imaging alone. The results challenged the rote use of ICP monitoring in the traumatic brain injured patient. A similar study has not been identified in the stroke population. In stroke patients, bedside neuromonitoring is supported by consensus guidelines.[10,11] Clear benefits of EVD monitoring in SAH are described.[6,36–38] Much of the controversy surrounding neuromonitoring of ischemic stroke centers on the usefulness of neuromonitoring in detecting delayed cerebral ischemia (DCI).[7,8,10–13,40]

A positive relationship between patient outcomes and the use of invasive neuromonitoring has been reported in the literature. In small cohort studies, improved outcomes in poor-grade SAH were reported when invasive neuromonitoring was initiated early in the course of treatment.[13] No outcome benefit with the use of invasive neuromonitoring was reported in patients with good-grade SAH who developed secondary deterioration due to DCI. However, a reduction of neuroimaging and transports were noted suggesting secondary benefits of invasive neuromonitoring in the subset of patients[13]

Intracranial monitoring is not without inherent risks.[8,36] The rate of infection in EVDs in the literature is variable prompting calls for standardized guidelines for maintenance.[27,35–37] Failure to act on data obtained is counterproductive. Reservations concerning the true benefit of the technology arise when failure to follow established guidelines is prevalent in clinical practice. This has been recognized as problematic in care rendered to the TBI patient.[41] Yuan and colleagues[42] reported ICP monitoring overall was not significantly superior to no ICP monitoring regarding mortality. Subgroup analysis of studies published after 2012 indicated an association between decreased mortality and patients with ICP monitors in place. The investigators suggested that standardized management and rigorous adherence to Brain Trauma Foundation guidelines may have been responsible for this finding. Although guidelines for the care of stroke patient exist, the paucity of guidelines for the use of multimodal monitoring in stroke patients is concerning.[11] Kieninger and colleagues[8] found that interventions to address pathologic values obtained during multimodal monitoring of patients with SAH did not occur in almost 50% of the participants in their study. This inaction was attributed to the absence of a clear algorithm for treatment.[8] Furthermore, a lack of controlled trials demonstrating the benefit of multimodal monitoring hinders recommendations for use in stroke patient.[16] A need for further research is indicated.

SUMMARY

Invasive neuromonitoring provides crucial data to guide the care of critically ill neuroscience patients. A variety of devices to monitor patients is available. Devices such as IPMs and EVDs are routinely used to detect and intervene in instances of increased ICP. Brain oxygenation levels are most frequently assessed with PbtO2 monitors. Metabolic changes in the brain are identified when cerebral microdialysis is introduced into the management plan. Each of these devices comes with its advantages and disadvantages. The decision regarding optimal device selection for a particular patient scenario is made based on thoughtful consideration of many factors.

Despite the unwavering reliance on ICP monitoring, the technology does not capture early ischemic changes and has limitations in the care of stroke patients. Advocates of multimodality monitoring cite the value of early detection of changes in brain oxygenation levels and brain metabolism as advantageous in optimizing patient outcomes. The data obtained from multimodal monitoring can be immense. The literature has demonstrated that integration of the data does not consistently occur.[5,8,20] An integrated system that collects and analyzes data as a whole, rather than individually, would allow for individualized treatment and optimal patient care. Such systems are not widely applied in the management of stroke.[18,20] As has been demonstrated, the impact of intracranial monitoring in the published literature is variable. The ultimate benefit of intracranial monitoring in patients with stroke, either alone or as a component of multimodal monitoring, is unknown. Further research to clarify the role of intracranial monitoring in the stroke population is needed.

CLINICS CARE POINTS

- The overarching goal of stroke management is to prevent secondary brain ischemia.
- Invasive neuromonitoring permits trending of ICP and monitoring of cerebral oxygentation and metabolism.

- Devices such as IPMs and EVDs are routinely used to detect and intervene in instances of increased ICP, most frequently in patients with SAH.
- ICP monitoring alone should not be the sole source of information on which therapy is guided but should be incorporated into the arsenal of emerging and promising invasive neuromonitoring devices.
- Multimodal monitoring is recommended to enhance stroke patient management by identifying early ischemic changes not detected with ICP monitoring alone.

DISCLOSURE

The author has nothing to disclose.

REFERENCES

1. Brain Trauma Foundation, American Association of Neurologic Surgeons, Congress of Neurologic Surgeons, et al. Guidelines for the management of severe traumatic brain injury VI: indications for intracranial pressure monitoring. J Neurotrauma 2007;24(Suppl 1):S37–44.
2. Chestnut R, Videtta W, Vespa P, et al. Intracranial pressure monitoring: Fundamental considerations and rationale for monitoring. Neurocrit Care 2014; 21(Suppl 2):S64–84.
3. Chen H, Stiefel M, Oddo M, et al. Detection of cerebral compromise with multimodality monitoring in patients with subarachnoid hemorrhage. Neurosurgery 2011; 69:53–63.
4. Olson D, Kofke W, O'Phelan K, et al. Global monitoring in the neurocritical care unit. Neurocrit Care 2015;22:333–47.
5. Fan J-L, Nogueira RC, Brassard P, et al. Integrative physiological assessment of cerebral hemodynamics and metabolism in acute ischemic stroke. J Cereb Blood Flow Metab 2021;423:454–70.
6. Censullo J, Firikh A, Mulkey M, et al. Nursing care of the patient with aneurysmal subarachnoid hemorrhage. AANN clinical practice guideline series. Glenview (IL): American Association of Neuroscience Nurses; 2018.
7. Veldeman M, Albanna W, Weiss M, et al. Invasive multimodal neuromonitoring in aneurysmal subarachnoid hemorrhage: a systematic review. Stroke 2021;52: 3624–32.
8. Kieninger M, Meichelbock K, Bele S, et al. Brain multimodality monitoring in patients suffering from acute aneurysmal subarachnoid hemorrhage: clinical value and complications. J Integ Neurosci 2021;20(3):703.
9. Michels DM, Van Dijk LC, Tavy DL. Perioperative stroke during carotid endarterectomy: benefits of multimodal neuromonitoring - a case report. BMC Neurol 2022;22. https://doi.org/10.1186/s12883-022-02835-7.
10. Le Roux P, Menon DK, Citerio G, et al. Consensus summary statement of the international multidisciplinary consensus conference on multimodality monitoring in neurocritical care. Neurocrit Care 2014;21(S2):1–26.
11. Kleindorfer DO, Towfighi A, Chaturvedi S, et al. 2021 guideline for the prevention of stroke in patients with stroke and transient ischemic attack: a guideline from the American Heart Association/American Stroke Association. Stroke 2021;52: e364–7.

12. Zhong W, Ji Z, Sun C. A review of monitoring methods for cerebral blood oxygen saturation. Healthcare 2021;9:1104.

13. Veldeman M, Albanna W, Weiss M, et al. Treatment of delayed cerebral ischemia in good-grade subarachnoid hemorrhage: a role for invasive neuromonitoring? Neurocrit Care 2021;35:172–83.

14. Kirkman MA, Smith M. Multimodal neuromonitoring. Anes Clin 2016;34(3): 511–23.

15. Yang Y, Chang T, Luo T. Multimodal monitoring for severe traumatic brain injury. Neurosurgery 2017;23:1346–9.

16. Tasneem N, Samaniego EA, Pieper C, et al. Brain multimodality monitoring: a new tool in neurocritical care of comatose patients. Crit Care Res Prac 2017. https://doi.org/10.1155/2017/6097265. Article ID 6097265.

17. Fiore M, Bogossian E, Creteur J, et al. Role of brain tissue oxygenation ($PbtO2$) in the management of subarachnoid haemorrhage: a scoping review protocol. BMJ Open 2020;10:e35521.

18. Goyal K, Khandelwal A, Kedia S. Multimodal neuromonitoring: current scenario in neurocritical care. J Neuroanaesthesiology Crit Care 2019;6(2):062–71.

19. Chestnut R, Temkin N, Carney N, et al. A trial of intracranial-pressure monitoring in traumatic brain injury. N Engl J Med 2012;367:2471–81.

20. Ruhatiya RS, Adukia SA, Manjunath RB, et al. Current status and recommendation in multimodal neuromonitoring. Indian J Crit Care Med 2020;24(5):353–60.

21. Livesay SL. The bedside nurse: the foundation of multimodal neuromonitoring. Crti Care Nurs Clin N Am 2016;28:1–8.

22. March K, Madden L. Intracranial pressure management. In: Littlejohns LR, Bader MK, editors. AACN-AANN protocols for practice: monitoring technologies in critically ill neuroscience patients. Sudbury (Ontario): Jones and Bartlett; 2009. p. 35–69.

23. Hinkle JL, Heck C. Monitoring for neurologic dysfunction. In: Booker KJ, editor. Critical care nursing: monitoring and treatment for advanced nursing practice. Ames (IA): Wiley Blackwell; 2015. p. 87–103.

24. Zrelak PA, Eigsti J, Fetzick A, et al. Evidence-based review: nursing care of adults with severe traumatic brain injury. AANN clinical practice guideline series. Glenview (IL): American Association of Neuroscience Nurses; 2020.

25. Greenberg SM, Ziai WC, Cordonnier C, et al. 2022 Guideline for the management of patients with spontaneous intracerebral hemorrhage: a guideline from the American Heart Association/American Stroke Association. Stroke 2022;53.

26. Lara LR, Puttgen HA. Multimodality monitoring in the neurocritical care unit. Continuum. Lifelong Learn Neurol 2018;24(6):1776–88.

27. Roh D, Park S. Brain multimodality monitoring: updated perspectives. Curr Neurol Neurosci Rep 2016;16:56.

28. Vinciguerra L, Bosel J. Noninvasive neuromonitoring: current utility in subarachnoid hemorrhage, traumatic brain injury, and stroke. Neurocrit Care 2017;27: 122–40.

29. Richter J, Sklienda P, Chatterjee N, et al. Elevated jugular venous oxygen saturation after cardiac arrest. Resuscitation 2021;169:214–9.

30. Oddo M, Hutchinson PJ. Understanding and monitoring brain injury: the role of cerebral microdialysis. Intensive Care Med 2018;44:1945–8.

31. Muralidharan R. External ventricular drains: management and complications. Surg Neurol Int 2015;6:S271–4.

32. Morone P, Dewan M, Zuckerman SL, et al. Craniometrics and ventricular access: a review of Kocher's, Kaufman's, Paine's, Menovksy's, Tubbs', Keen's, Frazier's, Dandy's, and Sanchez's Points. Oper Neurosurg 2020;18:461–9.

33. Greenberg MS. Operations and procedures. In: Handbook of neurosurgery. 7th edition. New York: Thieme; 2010. p. 207–14.

34. Leeper B, Lovasik D. Cerebrospinal drainage systems: external ventricular and lumbar drains. In: Littlejohns LR, Bader MK, editors. AACN-AANN protocols for practice: monitoring technologies in critically ill neuroscience patients. Sudbury (Ontario): Jones and Bartlett; 2009. p. 71–82.

35. Fried HI, Nathan BR, Rowe AS, et al. The insertion and management of external ventricular drains: an evidence-based consensus statement. Neurocrit Care 2016;24:61–81.

36. Rajshekhar V, Harbaugh RE. Results of routine ventriculostomy with external ventricular drainage for acute hydrocephalus following subarachnoid haemorrhage. Acta Neurochir 1992;115:8–14.

37. Hasan D, Vermeulen M, Wijdicks EF, et al. Management problems in acute hydrocephalus after subarachnoid hemorrhage. Stroke 1989;20:747–53.

38. Kuo LT, Huang AP-H. The pathogenesis of hydrocephalus following aneurysmal subarachnoid hemorrhage. Int J Mol Sci 2021;22:5050.

39. Vespa P, Menon D, LeRoux P, et al. Participants in the international multidisciplinary consensus conference on multimodality monitoring. The international multi-disciplinary consensus conference on multimodality monitoring: future directions and emerging technologies. Neurocrit Care 2014;21(Suppl 2):S270–81.

40. Okonkwo DO, Shutter LA, Moore C, et al. Brain oxygen optimization in severe traumatic brain injury phase-II: a phase II randomized trial. Crit Care Med 2017;45(11):1907–14.

41. Shafi S, Barnes SA, Millar D, et al. Suboptimal compliance with evidence-based guidelines in patients with traumatic brain injuries. J Neurosurg 2014;120.773–7.

42. Yuan Q, Xing W, Yirui S, et al. Impact of intracranial pressure monitoring on mortality in patients with traumatic brain injury: a systematic review and meta-analysis. J Neurosurg 2015;122:574–87.

Stroke Rehabilitation

Helen P. Neil, RN, MSN-HCSM, CLNC, FCN

KEYWORDS

- Stroke • Disability • Survival • Stroke rehabilitation • Post-stroke
- Post-stroke depression

KEY POINTS

- Stroke
- Stroke rehabilitation
- Post-stroke
- Post-stroke rehabilitation

INTRODUCTION

The Centers for Disease Control and Prevention (CDC) states someone in the United States has a stroke every 40 s and that stroke is a leading cause of severe long-term disability.[1] The American Heart Association (AHA) has reported that nearly 75% of stroke victims experience mild to moderate disability, and 15% to 30% experience severe disability following stroke.[2] Among post-stroke survivors, it is anticipated that greater than 20% experience constraints in activities of daily living (ADLs) and greater than 30 in instrumental ADL (IADLs).[2] Activities of daily living include self-care strategies, and instrumental activities of daily living are essential for the post-stroke survivor to be functional and live independently in their community, including driving, cooking, cleaning, and managing finances.[3]

Contemporary developments in acute stroke treatment and neurocritical care have increased the survival rates of stroke victims with varying degrees of disability.[4] The use of stroke-specific treatment modalities has contributed to the quality of life of stroke survivors and their families. Stroke recovery is a complicated biological and neurologic path with many factors influencing the improvement course, and a focus on neurorehabilitation optimizes rehabilitation outcomes.[5] Recovery is the extent to which a body structure and function return to the pre-stroke state, and rehabilitation includes interventions designed to regain the lost body functions.[6]

The Cost of Stroke

The Centers for Disease Control and Prevention (CDC) states that stroke-related costs in the United States came to nearly $53 billion between 2017 and 2018 (CDC, 2022).

Louisiana State University Health New Orleans, School of Nursing, 1900 Gravier Street Room 328, New Orleans, LA 70112, USA
E-mail address: hneil@lsuhsc.edu

Crit Care Nurs Clin N Am 35 (2023) 95–99
https://doi.org/10.1016/j.cnc.2022.11.002
ccnursing.theclinics.com

Abbreviations	
ADL	Activites of Daily Living
IADL	instrutmental Activities of Daily Living
PDS	Post-stroke Depression
NIHSS	National Institue of Health Stroke Score
BDI - II	Beck Depression Inventory II
FIM	Functional Independence Measure

Stroke imposes substantial financial burdens on individual, families, and society due to the morbidity and mortality.[7] Post-stroke depression is associated with longer acute care hospitalization, longer rehabilitation stays, and poorer rehabilitation outcomes. Post-stroke depression is often correlated with higher rates of suicidal ideation and stroke mortality.[8] Another factor that affects stroke costs is age; individuals > 65 years of age are usually covered by Medicare and are typically affected less financially. Individuals < 65 years of age may lose employment and insurance due to stroke disabilities and experience a huge impact on families financially. Stroke recurrence, prescription drug costs, long-term care costs, and nursing home costs impact a stroke survivors ability to meet financial needs. Increasing survival rates, type of stroke, age, and aggregate costs provide an estimate of lifetime cost of stroke; social workers and case managers on the stroke team can assist patients and families preparation for lifestyle changes.[7]

Stroke Rehabilitation

Stroke rehabilitation has been roughly defined as any aspect of stroke care that aims to reduce disability and promote participation in ADLs and IADLs to improve quality of life.[4] A comprehensive stroke rehabilitation program is essential to achieve a maximum level of independence for stroke survivors. Rehabilitation and education of the patient, family, and caregivers are vital components of the continuum of stroke care and should start as soon as possible.[5] Psychological care is also integral to stroke rehabilitation; post-stroke depression (PSD) is considered the most frequent and significant neuropsychiatric consequence of stroke that negatively affects stroke rehabilitation outcomes.[9]

Stroke rehabilitation focuses on reducing disability, preventing deterioration of function, and achieving the highest possible level of independence by treating the physical, cognitive, psychological, social, and vocational impairments. Post-stroke rehabilitation is a complicated, vigorous, and multifactorial process that includes genetic, pathophysiological, sociodemographic, neuropsychological, and therapeutic modalities that must be incorporated to achieve the patient's goals. Peak neurologic recovery occurs within the first 3 months of the initial insult, and rehabilitation is exceptionally beneficial to neurologic and functional recovery. Rehabilitation starts in the acute care setting, progresses to an inpatient acute rehabilitation setting, and continues post-discharge in an outpatient or home-based program. A significant part of the transition includes community access, access to support groups, vocation counseling, and peer interaction.[5]

Rehabilitation management begins with clinical assessments of the new limitations using standardized measurement instruments. Measuring the outcomes of health care interventions with standardized instruments is a central component of determining therapeutic effectiveness.[10] Assessments typically include a physiatrist, rehabilitation nursing, physical therapy, occupational therapy, speech therapy, recreational therapy, neuropsychology, social services, case managers, nutritional specialists, respiratory therapists, and vocational counselors.[5] The most frequently used instrument of measure for stroke patients is the National Institute of Health Stroke Scale (NIHSS); Lyden[11] refers to it as the gold standard. The NIHSS evaluates the level of consciousness, gaze, visual fields, facial palsy, arm and leg motor ability, ataxia, sensory, language, dysarthria, and neglect. The Functional Independence Measure (FIM) assesses six areas of function (self-care, sphincter control, transfers, locomotion, communication, and social cognition) and is widely used in stroke rehabilitation. The American Stroke Association conducted a study and found that the Beck Depression Inventory-II (BDI-II) instrument was reliable for measuring PSD.[12] The twenty-one-item BDI – II was developed to detect changes in depressive symptoms in mental health care settings.[13]

A comprehensive team approach to stroke rehabilitation is the most effective approach because it ensures communication between health care providers and allows for team members to work accommodatingly with the patient and family to reach maximum potential.[14] The team leader is a medical specialist such as a neurologist or physiatrist who is not responsible for the overall management of the patient's recovery during the rehabilitation phase. The rehabilitation nurse is the coordinator of all of the team members to develop an understanding of the patient's condition, progress, and desired disposition. In addition, the rehabilitation nurse takes all of the progress of each therapy session and incorporates it into their care. Each rehabilitation team requires a social worker, case manager, or rehab counselor to advise the patient and family on financial impacts, community resources, support groups, and outpatient needs. The physiotherapist assesses the stroke patient with mobility needs such as turning in the bed, transfers to a chair, standing, balance, and walking. The physical therapist will communicate with the team the safest way to transfer the patient as they progress during the program. Respiratory therapy coach's patients with cough and deep breathing exercises that can assist with prevention of respiratory infections. Respiratory therapy also plays a key role in assisting with weaning stroke patients during trach placement. The speech therapist assists patients with dysphagia, dysarthria, cognitive impairments, and communication. The speech therapist will communicate with the team on the best way to communicate with the patient and what level diet they may tolerate. The occupational therapist assesses and manages the effects of the stroke that affect self-care activities. Stroke patients need education for the patient and caregivers on the best methods to adapt to changed abilities by designing specific activities concentrating on the skills needed to return home. One of the most important events of the rehab experience is the home visit to determine which modifications are necessary to ensure a safe return. The neuropsychologist assesses the effect on memory, cognition, and emotional changes due to alterations in brain function. Neuropsychologists assess for post-stroke depression, treatment of behavior problems, counseling with family issues, and returning to the workforce[14]

Upon completion of the assessment, short-term and long-term goals are established in close collaboration between the patient, family, and health care professionals. Identifying a patient's goals is a crucial component of the success of the rehabilitation program.[15] Involving the patient and family increases motivation and fulfillment. The International Classification of Functioning, Disability, and Health (ICF) is used for goal setting by allowing the health care providers to map the specific targets for the appropriate intervention. The use of the ICF allows all members of the interprofessional rehabilitation team to use the same language. Research indicates that a patient's contribution and progress are more significant when goals focus on participation and less on physical ability.[15]

Depression screening and treatment are essential to every comprehensive stroke rehabilitation program due to compromised quality of life, diminished rehabilitation outcomes, gait recovery, and increased mortality.[16] Rehabilitation health care providers need to be aware of risk factors for PSD: low-level education, low socioeconomic status, increased severity of a stroke, less than six-five years of age, obesity, female, and decreased ability to perform self-care strategies.[16] Although PSD is typically associated with adverse outcomes, it is treatable; early detection and proper management are essential to obtain better rehabilitation outcomes for patients with PSD.[17]

SUMMARY

Despite contemporary rehabilitation strategies, stroke remains a leading cause of loss of function, limited mobility, psycho-social complications, and decreased quality of life. Stroke rehabilitation is a process that aims to prevent deterioration of function, increase function, and assist the patient in achieving the highest possible level of independence physically, socially, spiritually, psychologically, vocationally, and economically. The process begins with relearning activities of daily living such as grooming, bathing, toileting, eating, and dressing. As the patient progresses, stroke rehabilitation works on instrumental activities of daily living such as housekeeping, cooking, driving, and managing financial responsibilities.

The process of rehabilitation begins with interprofessional assessments and collaborative goal setting. During restoration and adaption, the patient and rehabilitation modify the goals to achieve maximum independence. The whole team works to assist the patient in achieving their goals. The physiatrist is the team leader that orders the treatment based on the team's suggestions:

- Physical therapists work on movement and balance.
- Occupational therapists assist with self-care strategies.
- Speech and language pathologist focuses on swallowing and communication deficits.
- Recreational therapies work on leisure activities to improve cognitive impairments.
- Neuropsychologists assist with the psycho-social complications associated with disability, isolation, and role changes.
- Social services work closely with case managers to ensure appropriate disposition with the necessary equipment to adapt to home life after stroke.
- Nutritional specialists develop diet considerations associated with swallowing and decreased risk of recurrent stroke.
- Vocational counselors assist with job training and placement.
- Rehabilitation nurses reinforce all aspects of therapeutic resources. Rehabilitation nurses are the cheerleaders when grooming is accomplished or the re-educator when safety measures are not followed. Rehabilitation nurses monitor for progress or regression and communicate with all team members.

Stroke rehabilitation is a complex process that involves multiple health care specialties and is the most efficient resource for a successful transition to home.[4]

REFERENCES

1. Tsao CW, Aday AW, Almarzooq ZI, et al. Heart disease and stroke statistics—2022 update: a report from the American Heart association. Circulation 2022; 145(8):e153–639.

2. Go AS, Mozaffarian D, Roger VL, et al. Heart disease and stroke statistics—2014 update: a report from the American Heart Association. Circulation 2014;129: e28–292.
3. Guo HJ, Sapra A. Instrumental activity of daily living. [Updated 2021 nov 21]. In: StatPearls [internet]. Treasure Island (FL): StatPearls Publishing; 2022.
4. Belagaje S. Stroke rehabilitation. Continuum (Minneap Minn) 2017;23(1):238–53.
5. Bagherpour R, Dykstra DD, Barrett AM, et al. A comprehensive neurorehabilitation program should be an integral part of a comprehensive stroke center—. Front Neurol 2014;5(27):1–5.
6. Stinear CM, Lang CE, Zeiler S, et al. Advances and challenges in stroke rehabilitation. Lancet Neurol 2020;19:349–60.
7. Taylor T, Davis P, Torner J, et al. Lifetime cost of stroke in the United States. Stroke 1996;27(9):1459–66.
8. Husaini B, Levine R, Sharp L, et al. Depression increases stroke hospitalization cost: an analysis of 17,010 stroke pateints in 2008 by race and gender. Stroke Res Treat 2013;8464329:1–7.
9. Shi Y, Yang D, Zeng Y, et al. Risk factors for post-stroke depression: a meta-analysis. Front Aging Neurosci 2017;9:218.
10. van der Putten JJ, Hobart JC, Freeman JA, et al. Measuring change in disability after inpatient rehabilitation: comparison of the responsiveness of the Barthel index and the functional independence measure. J Neurol Neurosurg Psychiatr 1999;66:480–4.
11. Lyden P. Using the national institute of health stroke scale: a cautionary tale. Stroke 2017;48(2):513–9.
12. Berg A, Lonnqvist J, Palomaki H, et al. Assessment of depression after stroke: a comparison of different screening instruments. Stroke 2009;40(2):523–9.
13. Turner A, Hambridge J, White H, et al. Depression screening in stroke: comparison of alternative measures with the structured diagnostic interview for the diagnostic and statistical manual of mental disorders, Fourth Edition (Major Depressive Episode) as the criterion standard. Stroke 2012;43:1000–5.
14. Stroke Recovery Association NSW. The Stroke Team. Reducing the impact of stroke. 2022. Available at: https://strokensw.org.au/about-stroke/initial-stroke-what-now/the-stroke-team/. Accessed August 8, 2022.
15. Preede L, Soberg H, Dalen H, et al. Rehabilitation goals and effects of goal achievement on outcome following an adapted physical activity-based rehabilitation intervention. Patient preference and adherence 2021;15:1545–55.
16. Park GY, Im S, Lee SJ, et al. The association between post-stroke depression and the activities of daily living/gait balance in patients with first-onset stroke patients—p. sychiatry Invest 2016;13(6):659–64.
17. Medeiros GC, Roy D, Kontos N, et al. Post-stroke depression: a 2020 updated review. Gen Hosp Psychiatry 2020;66:70–80.

Moving?

Make sure your subscription moves with you!

To notify us of your new address, find your **Clinics Account Number** (located on your mailing label above your name), and contact customer service at:

Email: journalscustomerservice-usa@elsevier.com

800-654-2452 (subscribers in the U.S. & Canada)
314-447-8871 (subscribers outside of the U.S. & Canada)

Fax number: 314-447-8029

Elsevier Health Sciences Division
Subscription Customer Service
3251 Riverport Lane
Maryland Heights, MO 63043

*To ensure uninterrupted delivery of your subscription, please notify us at least 4 weeks in advance of move.

Printed and bound by CPI Group (UK) Ltd, Croydon, CR0 4YY

03/10/2024

01040467-0012